LIVING WELL
SIX PILLARS FOR
LIVING YOUR BEST LIFE

By Greg Horn

Lighthouse Press
2741 Marina Circle
Lighthouse Point, FL 33064
www.Living-Well.com

Hardcover ISBN: 978-0-9825159-6-9

Softcover ISBN: 978-0-9825159-3-8

This book is printed on acid-free paper.

Printed in the United States of America

Table of Contents

Foreword

The book you are about to read will open new doors for you. It will allow you to design your own personal laboratory to discover the levers within your direct control to help you escape the feeling of fatigue and welcome the feelings of vitality and a sunnier perspective. As you experiment with Greg's ideas, I promise that you will feel like a more integrated human being and, in the process, invite in a truly elevated new chapter in your journey.

My name is Richard Rakowski. I am a long-time friend and colleague of Greg. I am an engineer, businessman, husband, father, investor, healthcare transformation advocate, entrepreneur, and perpetual and passionate student of life.

I am honored to begin your journey in *Living Well* by sharing a few thoughts with you. I have lived 64 years inside a highly eclectic personal and professional life that has resulted in four healthy and happy children, two grandchildren, a taste of business success, unending nourishment from non-stop learning, and the ability to free myself from the shackled legacy of my parents, who spent six years in three different Nazi concentration camps.

Through my journey, I have seen that all of us can easily fall prey to taking things that are truly miraculous for granted. This can include the birth of child, the limitless show of lights in the night sky, and the sheer engineering genius of a human body in operation. Fortunately, I have successfully faced a few challenges with my own mortality and still live with the fact that my brother was not so lucky. Said most simply, as I interact with this thing called "life", my own experience informs me in a way that I am humbled, awed, and profoundly interested in the activity and patterns of our lives as we live them through our social, biological, and spiritual identities.

Despite the fact we have siloed the definition of our challenges into the realms of medicine, religion, and social repair, we are not fragmented beings: we are whole and integrated beings. Our feelings and moods affect our biology, and our biology affects our emotions. Our social and spiritual connectedness are tied to our immune system, and the root causes of our many and growing number of diseases cannot be isolated with a blood test or CT scan.

Yes, we are integrated beings with physical, spiritual, and emotional aspects. Any disturbance to any one of these three aspects is linked to and affects the other two. If we lose a long-time and beloved spouse, we run large risks of an untimely death. If we have a fight with our children, spouses, or neighbors, we can find ourselves in a mindless binge with Oreos, nachos, or rocky road ice cream. Loneliness and isolation are gateways to multiple cocktails, sleepless nights, and lethargy. Obesity drives self-esteem issues that, in turn, drive a loss of faith in matters of the flesh and spirit. We are a complete being with three aspects in harmony (or disharmony) with one another. That is a profound truth.

Most of us are very busy. Even more of us have become stressed with the pressures of the lives we inhabit. Things are moving very quickly, and we all sense that the role of cell phones, social media, and the rest of technology in our daily lives has become a dopamine-riddled addiction. Our work hours, childcare concerns, and commuting responsibilities are often in excess of the light within us to sustain our sense of balance, optimism, and self-awareness. All too often, the stress, speed, and lack of sleep force us into a pattern that is very difficult to escape. This pattern can manifest in corrosive nutrition, activities, and social behaviors that are all too easy to fall prey to and forge the scaffolding and compass of how we live our day-to-day lives. And yes, money problems are also a reliable ingredient of sleepless nights, marital incoherence, high blood pressure, clinical depression, and a sense of malaise/helplessness.

Many of us drink five cups of coffee each day to fight off fatigue, while at night we take a sleeping pill to accelerate the path to our ever-declining need to rest and dream. We eat while we work and mindlessly eat while we drive to and from work. We take over-the-counter and prescription medications to soothe the daily effects of the narrative of our lives. It is no surprise that many of us complain of fatigue, while others lament that there is simply no time for the morning walk or 45 minutes in the gym. Then, of course, we impose judgment and guilt on ourselves for skipping our needed activity.

From time to time, just like you and everyone else, I find myself inside many, if not all, of these challenges. Precious few people walking this planet are immune to the realities of life. The trick is to face those realities with increasingly effective tools.

While more than enough negative outside influences are beyond our control to explain our many challenges, we also have confirming moments in our lives where we can author a shift in our whole selves. These are the moments that we take the reins as a scientist in our laboratory and successfully experiment with those things we can control and influence.

I have come to believe that in a metaphorical sense, each of us can live a part of our lives as both a laboratory scientist and the specimen that the scientist studies. We have an opportunity to experiment with different ideas, techniques, and approaches that result in greater well-being, increased energy, and happiness. Each of us is different, so the laboratory is deeply personal and individualized. I have been experimenting for over 50 years and realize that it's ok to be just a little curious about what might happen if we consciously observe what happens to our mood, sleep, and energy when we add or subtract sugar, exercise, and stress.

From my own direct experience, I have come to believe that shifting a few simple parts of my day can result in a dramatic move from fatigue to vitality, insecurity to confidence, darkness to light. I also have seen how my own behavior with food, sleep, and exercise can shift my sense that the world is riddled with scarcity to a world that is full of hope and abundance.

I have found that the rewards for living in alignment with my true self have a rapid impact in less than five days. This impact begins to create a self-sustaining engine.

I am bolstered by evidence all around me of people who take an all-too-infrequent break from their corrosive lives to participate in an experience that provides evidence of the natural innate potential residing within them for a better life. These times may come from indulging in a massage while visiting a spa. It might come from making love or watching children in glee as they conquer a fear that has consumed and paralyzed their potential. It might come from the simple but powerful ritual of an unrushed candlelight dinner and a glass of wine with someone who cares about us and our feelings as we engage in conversation that reminds us of our humanity and social essence. All of these snapshot experiences reveal our true nature and our ability to live well. All of these things, and more, can provide evidence that lying within us are the road map and rewards of living well.

Over these many years, my little laboratory of one has revealed that even the smallest catalyst or change can unlock larger aspects of my whole self on the road to living well. The catalyst can begin with the most simple of self-authored changes that influence and cascade into other aspects of our daily lives. Improved sleep, nutrition, and activity have a predictable and almost immediate impact on our emotions and self-esteem. People in our orbit begin to see and sense a change in us when we shift toward living well and, in the process, they can't help themselves and provide positive feedback that helps propel and accelerate that change. There is simple but great power in someone noticing that you have changed for the better. It is a potent and healthy drug.

This point of view, based on my deep personal experience and a career creating and transforming health care companies, leads me to my friend and colleague, Greg Horn.

Greg Horn has been three things in my life. First and foremost, he is a stalwart (old school) kind of friend who can be relied upon 24/7 for his heart, attention, and insight. I cherish the 20-plus-year gift of his friendship. Second, he has also been a business colleague and partner when he led GNC and other nutritional business ventures. I have been privileged to see him work and align his values with every decision and action he takes in an often-challenging world of business. Finally, I have been a student of his journey through a severe health challenge that he overcame with unusual focus, perseverance, and insight. It is this insight that forms the basis of *Living Well*.

I hope you enjoy what you are about to read and derive great value from the words to follow. Please take comfort in the fact that all of us are nothing more than porous beings who absorb the increasingly challenging and stressful environment where we live. In that light, it is no surprise that we struggle. So I ask that in that light, you be open, kind, and forgiving with yourself. I am honored and pleased to say that this over-arching environment now includes Greg Horn and the road map of opportunity he constructed to "live well."

Humbly,

Richard Rakowski

Living Well: My Story

I wrote this book to help you live a better life.

Over the past couple of decades, I've learned a lot about living well. I've been fortunate to have access to the world's leading experts in nutrition, exercise, sleep, and evolutionary biology. I've served as CEO for both the most successful vitamin retailer and the most successful health food supplement brand. Along the way, I've been seriously sick with a condition from which most people never recover. I've recovered my health and learned to live a very full life in good health. In short, I've learned a lot of this the hard way and have been very lucky.

And I want to share what I've learned.

I will share positive actions that can lead to dramatic changes in your health and how you feel, perform, look, and enjoy life. How to eat for health, exercise for life, and sleep like an animal.

Most importantly, I want to share the science behind the art of living well.

Everything in this book is backed by published research, unless I specifically note that something is my own theory or experience. That's important, because while many areas of health and wellness are backed by research, it's still a young field, and new findings often dispel earlier opinions and assumptions. I bring the science, with references when I can, so you don't have to take anything on faith.

The benefits from applying these insights are remarkable, tangible, and critical for getting the most out of life.

This book can help you live your best life. What could be more important than that?

As a teenager, I had an epiphany. I was exactly 15-1/2 the winter I figured out what I wanted to do when I grew up. The half-year is important, because for the first half of my 15th year, I was a typical teenager. I ate at fast food joints. I drank lots of soda. I ate sugary cereal for breakfast, candy after school, and ice cream for dessert.

Then I read an old paperback, a book that had been on my mom's bookshelf for years. The book was *Sugar Blues* by William Dufty[1], and it described how addicted we were to sugar and the impact it had on our health. I had never really made the connection between diet and health before, and I was intrigued. So, I did an experiment and cut most sugar out of my diet for 10 days. The first couple of days were rough. But then…what a difference! The way I felt, my energy level, my mental clarity, and how I performed physically were radically better. It was such a visceral connection to something so life-improving and previously undiscovered (at least to my 15-year-old self) that I was smitten.

With the zeal and surety reserved for the almost totally naïve, I decided to learn everything I could about the connection between what we do with our bodies and how we feel, look, and perform. Mostly for selfish reasons at first, I decided to become an expert at the art of living.

I knew what I wanted to do when I grew up: I wanted to live well.

Ever since then (30-plus years and counting), I've been obsessively reading and experimenting with everything I can get my hands on about diet, nutrition, exercise, sleep, attitude, and daily activities and their connection to health and their role in living the best life possible. I've relentlessly sought out, met, and even worked professionally with the leading scientists in each of these fields, collaborating with some of them to advance the science and create new commercial applications for their insights and inventions. I've created healthy living and nutrition products and brands that work and now sell over $1 billion per year. And I've loved almost every minute of it.

Through a combination of early focus, great timing, and good luck, my second job out of graduate school was to create a set of credible nutrition product brands for retailer GNC. For me, this was the job of my dreams. I was so enthused about the potential to bring effective nutrition products to the people who could benefit the most that I worked six to seven days a week for almost a decade. (At the office, as this was before telecommuting or the Internet.) By the time I was 30, GNC was a billion-dollar company, and I was overseeing all the sales and marketing. During this period, I developed and launched GNC's core brand message of "Live Well," with the strong belief that enabling people to live well was the real purpose of the health and fitness industry. By age 36, I became the CEO. I was on top, running the largest health and nutrition company in the world and selling brands I had created in the category I had wanted to lead since age 15. We even changed the GNC logo to include "Live Well".

Then I got sick. Maybe it was the new office building, with new carpets, flame-retardant-soaked paneling and furniture, and recirculating air. Maybe it was when I was in a bus crash, where scores of fluorescent lights burst and filled the air with mercury vapor and phosphors. Maybe it was some natural predisposition that would have happened anyway. But I was sick. At first, I thought it was stress, or perhaps just premature aging, because when I took a rare vacation and was outdoors, I felt dramatically better after only a few days. But when I returned to the office, I was sick again almost instantly. Not only were my muscles stiff and achy, but I also suffered from blurred vision and dull headaches. I had a loss of concentration, and my usually very high energy level was gone. These symptoms would all come back almost immediately upon returning to my beautiful corner office.

Eventually, my ailment was diagnosed as multiple chemical sensitivities (or MCS), a little-understood condition that many doctors still think is "all in your head." It's not. It's very real. It happens to people who come back into their homes too soon after termite tenting, to chemotherapy patients, and to chemical workers. The general perception is that there's not much you can do, and it only gets worse. Eventually you won't be able leave the house, work at an office job, or have many normal relationships. That didn't sound too good to me, and I wanted to avoid that progression by applying my exposure to the difference a lifestyle can make for health.

I decided to take radical action. To start, I negotiated a friendly exit from the job of my dreams. I moved to a climate where there would be lots of fresh air year round. Luckily, my brilliant wife Laura and I were able to build a house from scratch using only clean materials and with about one-third of the covered living space outdoors. I changed my furniture, especially my mattress, to an organic cotton version without the chemicals found in traditional mattresses. I rented office space and remodeled it to be clean and safe. I stepped up my exercise and changed my diet to mostly organic foods. I reached out to experts in a wide range of health fields and learned even more.

And I got better. My energy came back. My thoughts cleared. My body healed, and the spring returned to my step.

But I didn't have a job. And at that time, I couldn't even walk into most offices without having a serious relapse. For more than two years, I basically couldn't work indoors in case new carpet or furniture was in the office building.

That was the beginning of my entrepreneurial career.

Deciding what to do next did not take long. By now, the connection between nutrition and health that first enthralled me as a teenager was clear to many, and the science was evolving to the point where it was easy to see nutrition moving closer to real medicine. I would simply continue doing what I loved by expanding my knowledge of nutrition and health and building new brands combining effective and clinically proven nutrition therapies marketed as consumer products. Working with the leading scientists and innovators in the fields of health, food, and nutrition to commercialize innovations has turned out to be a fascinating, rewarding, and profitable field of specialization for more than a decade. With new validation and discoveries emerging daily at the frontiers of health and nutrition, the field promises to have a continued fascination and positive impact on health for decades to come.

Over the past couple of decades, I've been in hundreds of GNC and health food stores and heard from thousands of people just like you. They almost always tell me the same thing: They don't have enough energy; they feel foggy, creaky, and tired; they are stressed out with no time to work out or eat right; they are trying to lose weight; they want to feel better – they want to live well. This book is dedicated to them.

This book contains what I've learned after having continuous access to the world's leading experts in health and nutrition for almost three decades. After helping to build and then run two of the largest and most successful healthy living companies in the world. After being sick and learning how to recover. After striving to put it all together and live my own best life. Some of it is simple, things your grandmother told you. Some flies in the face of conventional wisdom, and some is downright surprising.

All of it works.

Let's get started.

Living Well: The Program

We are the products of more than a million years of human evolution, yet we live in a modern world that can be at odds with the way our bodies evolved. Our ancestors adapted in specific ways to respond to food, exercise, even the light of day. Over hundreds of generations, these adaptations shaped our bodies, brains, and consciousness to help us survive and thrive. However, over the course of just a few decades, we have radically altered our existence with electric lights, labor-saving machines, environmental chemicals, modern agriculture, highly processed food, computers, and numerous other developments. Many of these advancements, such as medicine, vaccines, and widely available foods have helped us live longer, safer, more stable lives. However, by and large, we are living an existence very different from the conditions that caused our bodies to evolve, and this has many negative effects on our health and well-being.

In creating the Living Well Program, I explored the disconnect between our modern living conditions and what has been encoded in our body through a million years of

evolution. As they say, "You don't know where you're going if you don't know where you've been." At the same time, it's also important to embrace what is good about modern life rather than trying to artificially recreate an idealized past. We're very fortunate to live in a time where the opportunities for a good life are available to more people than ever before in our history. To really live our best lives, we need to take advantage of the benefits of our modern world while understanding that the foundations of our bodies are largely the same as they were 10,000 years ago, and sometimes we need to accommodate the genes that got us here.

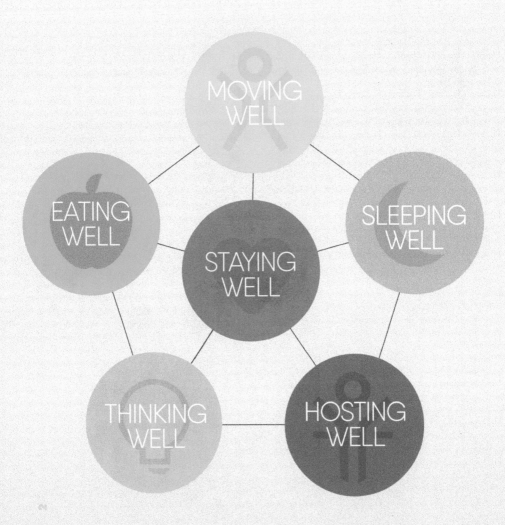

SIX PILLARS OF LIVING WELL

"For every complex problem there is a solution
that is simple, neat, and wrong."

—H. L. Mencken

Our culture seems to love simple, one-dimensional answers to questions about health, fitness, weight loss, and living well. I've read many books that promise if I just eat the right ratio of fat to carbs, or cut out grains, or do a simple 15-minute exercise program, that I can achieve my weight or fitness goals. My guess is that you have read some of these books too.

The problem with these simple solutions is that our bodies are complex, self-regulating organisms with multiple needs. The human genome has about 22,000 protein-coding genes,[2] and many of these genes can be turned on or off based on our diet, exercise, sleep patterns, exposure to nutrients and chemicals—even our exposure to light.[3] Any solution that hopes to address how to achieve good health and fitness must consider a variety of factors beyond just diet or exercise. Fortunately, the majority of these answers fit in with what we've long known about living well—get enough sleep, eat right, get some exercise—but with strong science to validate those observations and clarify what is really important and give us guidelines to follow.

In this book, I examine the Six Pillars of Living Well.
1. Thinking Well
2. Eating Well
3. Moving Well
4. Sleeping Well
5. Hosting Well
6. Staying Well

Some of these concepts are easy to understand—you can't live well unless you sleep and eat well. Others are less obvious, but no less important. Putting all Six Pillars to work will help you customize a program to help you live your best life, starting today.

Customizing the Living Well Program

This is not a one-size-fits-all program. Every person has a unique set of goals and definition of living well, so the Living Well Program is designed for customization. Read the recommendations, understand the science, and see how they apply to your own life. We must all make our own health decisions since we are the ones who must live with the results.

I think that every one of the Pillars is practical and important. However, you may not be ready to adopt all of them. Some can be incorporated into your life in a more gradual pace that's easier to accommodate. Every change will help you live a better life.

This is not a rigorous all-or-nothing program. Do what you can. Try new recommendations as you can. If you don't reach your goals one day—say you miss your exercise or break down and eat some junk food—let it go. Every day is a new chance to do a little better. It is important to make a commitment to your health, fitness and living well goals, but there's no need to beat yourself up over missing the mark—punishing yourself is not living well. Forgive and move on. In my experience, the "85% Rule" works best: About 85% is the right level of compliance with any health and diet regimen for long-term compliance. That ratio produces long-term results while eliminating worry and compulsion.

Enjoy this book and use it to help you better enjoy your life. If you're not enjoying life, you're not Living Well.

THINKING WELL

"Our goals can only be reached through a vehicle of a plan, in which we must fervently believe, and upon which we must vigorously act. There is no other route to success."

—*Pablo Picasso*

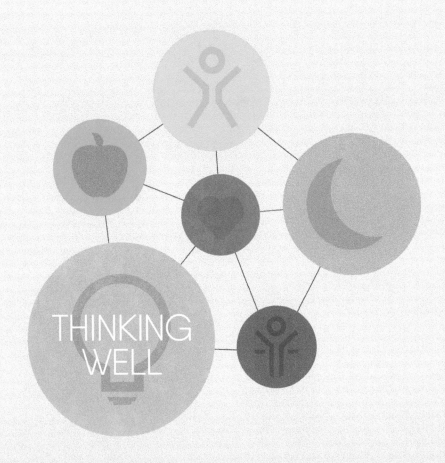

THINKING
WELL

THINKING WELL

My journey toward Living Well started with an epiphany at age 15-1/2. It turned a new direction when my life took an unexpected detour from a debilitating illness. Everyone's story is unique, but whatever brings you to the realization that you need to make a commitment to living well, you are here, reading this book.

In my first book, *Living Green*, I open the first chapter with this Chinese proverb: *"A journey of a thousand miles starts with a single step."* I've always found inspiration in that idea, and it has helped give me the courage to tackle challenges that seemed monumental at the outset. And while this proverb is true enough, **in reality, the journey begins with the decision to take the journey.**

If you've decided to start living well, this book is for you. It can be a road map and instruction manual along the way. To get where you want to be, however, will take some work. Let's face it, if the goals were easy to achieve, you'd have done them already.

The Power of Planning

I believe deeply in the power of planning and organization as a way to achieve goals. The person with the plan at least knows what they want and has an idea of how to achieve it. So while looking at planning and making task lists may initially seem out of place in a book about living well, this is the place to start. Why? Because it's very likely that what is holding you back from living the life you want isn't just a lack of research about what changes will make the most impact in your life. At some level, most everyone is aware that more sleep, more exercise, and a better diet would lead to health, weight, and fitness improvements. What's holding back a lot of people is the difficulty in juggling schedules and priorities to make time for these changes. This is why planning is key: it lets you figure out what is important in terms of reaching your objectives, and it helps make sure you do those important things. Along the way, good planning, prioritizing, and progress tracking helps you get more done overall as well. These are the kinds of changes that will make possible all the other changes you want to make in your life.

Before you can get started on your journey, you need to have some idea of where you are going. What does living well mean to you? Is it improving your health? Is it weight loss or better fitness? Reduced stress, improved relationships, a better career? Take time to think about your goals. Envision yourself living well—whatever that means to you.

Start now, right here in this book. You'll find a place to record your vision and goals on the next page. So grab a pencil and write down details from this vision. You can be as specific as you like, but give yourself a destination to aim toward. For example, "When I think of myself living well, I imagine having time and energy to spend with my kids. Being in good health and at a weight that makes me feel good. I have time to read books and exercise, and I'm doing well at work." Include what you like, leave out what you don't care about, and don't exceed one page.

Your aims will evolve over time, so *write your goals in pencil, not pen*. You may start out saying that you want to lose weight and modify that later to a specific weight you hope to reach. And after reading this book, you may modify your goals as you learn something new and compelling that alters your viewpoint. Perhaps six months from now, when you've accomplished some of your goals, you set new ones. Updating your goals isn't abandoning them. It means that you are incorporating new information and learning more about what is important to you.

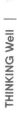

You can achieve the vision you just created of what your life looks like when you're living well. Set your mind to it, let it guide your daily decisions, keep doing it, and you can get there. This book will give you the tools to help you make informed decisions about how you can reach your goals. But even with the information, *you* still need to do it.

The Price of Progress

I am going to suggest some very positive actions you may want to take. These are based on not only science and but also direct experience from a lifetime in the field learning from leading researchers and people like you. These are actions I've taken myself, and I've seen them work for many others. But all progress comes at a price. You will need to make some decisions and stick with them if you expect to see changes. That price is often in time or commitment. The rewards for living your best life are immense, so I encourage you to figure out the price. Perhaps it's lost time in front of the TV in favor of a fitter, more energized body. Then pay that price.

Change is rarely comfortable. Even positive decisions—such as exchanging four hours of daily TV-watching for extra sleep, exercise, and social time—may still feel hard to actually do in the beginning or on challenging days. Setting goals and envisioning the rewards can help you stay focused.

To live your best life, you will have to practice what I call "generous selfishness" and protect your health. Being selfish in this way does not mean being anti-social or petty with your time. By selfishly guarding the time and priority you give your health, fitness, nutrition, and sleep, you will be generously protecting those who love you and rely on you. Maybe you are providing for a family. Maybe you have children or parents who rely on your care. Maybe you just have people who love you and want to spend time with you. Your ability to do all of these things depends on your health. This is fundamental to life and relationships: You will be a better father, mother, friend, leader, caregiver, and worker if you are living well. The opposite is also true. So, being selfish about protecting your health is actually, in my view, a form of generosity to those who rely on you and care about you.

As you think about living your best life and the actions you'll need to take to get there, understand that there will be costs. If you want to get a college degree or master's degree, you have to go to classes and study—you'll be giving up a lot. The same is true with losing weight, restoring your energy, regaining fitness, and improving your health. The rewards are great, but there will be a cost. As you consider each goal you've set, think about what you are willing to give up to reach that goal. Goals are more rewarding and long lasting when you accept the cost.

Your goals help by pointing you in the direction you want to go, but actually getting there takes action. I've found that writing down what you want to do—and often what you have done—can help accomplish these tasks much more efficiently. Whether you keep it loose or go into great detail, taking some time each day to write down a list of what you want to accomplish on that particular day is a great practice. (Being able to check things off once they're done can also be a great practice to reinforce that *you can do this.)*

I start each day by revising a list of what I need to do, sorted by importance. I've found this task list to be a key to keeping myself focused when things get hectic. It's also another source of satisfaction when I get to cross something off the list. It's fine to mix big, challenging tasks with small ones that are easily accomplished. Whether you use a piece of paper as I do, your computer scheduler, or a smartphone app, the act of distilling your tasks into a list can give you focus and motivate you to be more productive.

Not all tasks are of equal importance. When you're working with your list of daily tasks, take a moment to figure out what is really important. Which items on your list *must* get done? Once you figure those out, put a star by them and *do them first.*

When you do your hardest or most important tasks first in the day, it ensures you'll get them done with your most energy and focus. You'll also avoid procrastination.

Is there something on your list that you dread? Then that's the thing you need to put first. Typically, we tend to delay the things we dread or dislike. This sets up the pattern of checking email, replying to a few letters, or doing any of a number of low-priority tasks to avoid the harder ones. It's easy to fool ourselves into thinking that we're checking things off our task lists, but we're really killing time. This is a recipe for suddenly realizing in shock that it's noon and you haven't accomplished any of the things you really should have done.

Invariably, the tasks we dread are important ones. (Because if you don't like it, and if it isn't important, then why are you doing it at all?) Tackle these first. Get them done. You'll go into the rest of your day with a feeling of great accomplishment because of all you got done already. This is one of the reasons why I'm a big fan of exercising first thing in the morning—then it's out of the way, and I don't have to spend any time worrying about it. Plus, doing it feels great.

And once you finish that important task, what should you do next? That's right…probably the next-most-important task on your list. Do this and, at the end of the day, even if it turned out to be one of those days when you can't possibly accomplish everything, at least you will have knocked out the most important things. And you will have given them your best focus and energy, because you did them first.

Putting the Important things first also works in the microcosm. If you're exercising and you really want to get a strong core but hate abs exercises, put those first in your workout. You'll be done and free to move on to what you like better, and you will have given your full energy to where your priorities lie.

Track Your Progress

Tracking your progress is just as important as listing your tasks. For example, if you are doing an exercise program to reach a fitness goal, you'll find that writing down your progress on each exercise day helps keep you more motivated. For people trying to lose weight, *simply writing down everything you eat has been shown to be a highly effective weight loss tool, even if you're not actually dieting!*[4]

Several studies have shown that when a person writes down the foods they eat regularly, they lose more weight than those who don't keep a food diary. A study performed at Kaiser Permanente's Center for Health Research and published in 2008 found that the more the subjects tracked the foods they ate, the more weight they lost.[5] While this is a great tip if you want to lose some weight, I mention it here because I think it applies to the progress improvement you can see in any goal you undertake by writing down your actions and accomplishments. Weight loss is just a convenient way to measure the effect of this over long periods of time for challenging goals.

Journaling your progress keeps it in the forefront of your mind. In the case of food, people who track their food consumption in a food journal are more aware of the food they eat. This awareness makes it easier to maintain controls during tough times and feel the reward of sticking with their goals. Tracking exercise progress has a similar effect, in my experience.

People have long debated whether it's better to measure progress frequently or occasionally. Some believe that it's better not to focus too much on tracking progress, because it could make people obsessive (especially about goals like weight loss). Others argue that consistent monitoring is more effective, because it maintains awareness. In fact, research in this field indicates that *frequent monitoring is far more effective than occasional monitoring.*

Two independent studies published in 2013 looked at whether dieters would lose more weight by stepping on the scale every day compared to less frequent measurement. In both studies (one published in *Obesity*, the other in *Health*

Psychology), the daily weighing group lost significantly more weight. In the *Obesity* study, the more often a subject weighed himself, the more weight he or she lost (statistically).[6] In the *Health Psychology* study, not only did those who weighed themselves daily lose far more weight, but they continued to lose weight throughout the six-month study, whereas those who weighed themselves less frequently stalled out after the first few months.[7]   So consistent, frequent monitoring leads not only to faster progress, but longer-term progress—at least where weight loss is concerned.

I believe that this is true of most goals. In this example, weight loss was the topic because a lot more studies have been done in that area. Tracking your progress and measuring your outcomes *frequently* leads to better, faster, and more consistent progress.[8] I harness the "power of writing it down" every day and recommend that you try this as a way to maximize your effectiveness. Some goals don't lend themselves to stepping on a scale or writing down how many laps you swam or how far you walked, but you can still list the things you accomplished at the end of the day. If your vision of living well includes deepening your family relationships, there's no easy metric you can track. But you could certainly note that you called your mom that day and perhaps what you talked about. Jotting down these actions still helps keep your goal at the forefront of your mind and regularly reminds you of your progress. Combined with your morning task list, this journaling will keep you conscious of your tasks and accomplishments. I also find that writing down my accomplishments at the end of the day helps me sleep without obsessing over what I need to do the next day, and helps to close out my day with a sense of accomplishment.

Multi-Tasking Is a Lie

Modern life can be extremely distracting if you let it be—and maybe even if you don't let it. The constant updates from email, phone calls, social media, and all those interesting videos and articles that friends keep recommending can really put a drain on your focus. Add TV and video or digital games to the picture, and the constant exposure to digital stimuli can be overwhelming.

As a result, we are constantly inundated with distractions. Many of us call this "multi-tasking" but in reality, the research says that there is no multi-tasking. Computers may have multiple processors, but human beings can only concentrate on one thing at a time. What people call multi-tasking is actually switching between tasks quickly without getting as much done in a given time period. This is a terribly inefficient practice. It takes time to regain your focus each time you are interrupted from your task or you switch tasks.

People who try to multi-task have also been found to be distracted more easily than those who work on one thing at a time. A study published in *Journal of Experimental*

Psychology: Human Perception and Performance found that test subjects lost time every time they switched between tasks, and the more complex the tasks, the more time they lost.[9]

Beyond the time lost on any one activity, this constant onslaught of cell phone vibrations, messages, Internet media, web videos, and social media create a constant state of anxiety and distraction. As we acclimate to this level of constant stimulation, we crave it—constantly checking for messages in a vicious circle of distraction. Like the famous frog in the pot who is gradually warmed to a boil, we don't easily perceive how bad our life has become while we're in the middle of it.

I strongly recommend a "digital detox," a vacation from cell phones, social media, websites, twitter, TV, and any other form of digital entertainment. If this sounds like a shocking idea—something impossible to actually do – then that's a great indication that you may desperately need one. Ironically, if you feel that going without all these devices for a week would be a piece of cake, then you may not need a digital detox. This practice is gaining popularity in crowded and stressed-out cities like Tokyo and Korea, where "forest bathing" (spending time in forests) is actually prescribed by some psychologists for their patients.[10] And the research is building that social media overload has negative effects on mental health.[11]

Try it for a few days over a weekend, then for a week. Stop using the Internet, social media, and the rest. (You may want to post a status message saying that you're taking a week off from the Internet so people don't worry that you were abducted.) If your work requires email access, limit it to one session of reading and answering emails per day.

The first thing you're likely to learn is how hard this can be. You may initially get a new appreciation for how much you were hooked on digital device stimulation. However, after a week of adjusting to an existence less fraught with constant pings and buzzes, many people report feeling less distracted and more productive.

After you've completed a digital detox, you may want to keep up your regained focus with a weekly digital day off. A digital day off is a one-day mini-digital detox without any devices or email. Saturdays and Sundays make terrific digital days off. This lets you set aside the constant hum of digital life to focus on what is really around you. For me, a digital day off each week lets me retune my focus.

Email, text messages, and social media feeds come in at a constant and often relentless rate. If you tackled each one as it arrived, you might never get anything else done. Unless you are working in a job or on a project where a few minutes' lag in information could make or break you (most people don't, even if we'd like to think we do), then close your email browser, IM, and text message window most of the time and schedule three to four times of the day to check them. I recommend mid-morning, after you've accomplished something important on your task list, a couple of hours before the end of the day, and then just before you leave work or shut down for the day. Beyond that, don't let yourself lose focus just because someone else sent you an email or text message.

If you have a smart phone, disable "push" messaging so that you don't get buzzed every time someone sends you a message. This way you'll only see messages when you decide to check for them. The same goes for text messages and instant messaging. And turn off your phone at night. The people who regularly text and email you will come to understand that you don't instantly answer, and you will get a lot more productive time to work (and think) without distractions.

Starting with the Positive

Every morning, right when I wake up and before getting out of bed, I keep my eyes closed and spend a few minutes in that space between being asleep and awake thinking about the many things I'm grateful for in life. Call it a meditation, a gratitude exercise, an affirmation, or counting my blessings, this simple habit starts my day off on a very positive note.

It turns out this habit is also validated by research.

This may seem a little "softer" than the rest of the advice in this book, but it's based on solid science. Matthieu Ricard, a Buddhist monk (and also a biotechnologist by training), suggests that two opposing thoughts cannot occupy our minds at the same time. As an example, we can't shake hands and concurrently deliver a blow with those hands. Thus, by replacing anger, jealousy, or spite, we can train our minds to consciously replace those thoughts with acceptance, generosity, or forgiveness. Here again, science from universities in Madison, Wisconsin, and Berkeley, California, has validated this opinion. Monks from Ricard's order who had done thousands of hours of mind training and meditation tested four standard deviations higher than the average on a brain-scan measure of happiness when they meditated on "compassion."[12] This measurement is basically off the bell curve.

So staying positive from the moment we wake up can have a measurable impact on our brain waves and on the quality of the rest of our day.

PRESCRIPTION №1

1. Get Clear About Where You Want From Life

2. Set Priorities and Accept the Price

3. Practice "Generous Selfishness"

4. First Things First

5. Reclaim Your Focus with a Digital Detox

6. Don't Pretend to "Multi-Task"

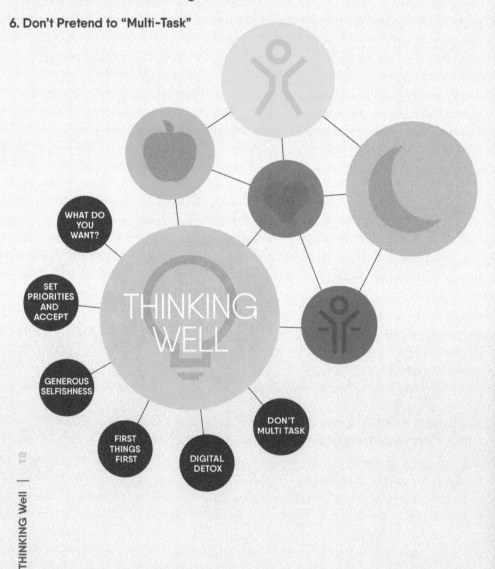

Prescription for Thinking Well

Thinking Well is the critically important first step toward living your best life, clarifying what you really want out of life, and freeing up the time and energy to get there. Like many things in life, taking back control of your time, focus, and mental energy starts with decisions reinforced by everyday habits:

1. Get Clear About Where You Want to Be in Life

Getting clear is a simple but incredibly powerful step toward Living Well. This can be as easy as setting one big goal, such as "Get healthier and lose 15 pounds by summer." Or you might be charting a more comprehensive course across many facets of life, including health, career, family, and contributions to society. A powerful benefit occurs when you commit your goals to paper, even if you never show anyone else. Write down what you want out of life as specifically as you can, starting with a single sentence, and do not exceed a single page of goals. I carry my piece of paper in my briefcase, check it often, and update it once a year, before the New Year's Eve party). It is highly rewarding and sometimes humbling to see where I've made progress. If it doesn't feel great to visualize what you've written, you're not clear yet. So keep writing! Getting clear should feel fantastic, and writing it down helps you make your vision tangible and even palpable.

2. Set Priorities and Accept the Price

Even Superman can't leap over tall buildings in a single bound, outrace a speeding bullet, and stop a train, ALL AT THE SAME TIME. Once you're clear on your goal(s), setting priorities is what will guide those goals to reality. If you want to get a book published as an author (as I do), for example, that goal will dictate the way you spend a good chunk of your time each day. It will mean rescheduling your meal, workout, and sleep times and taking less overtime at your day job. Those are big tradeoffs, and it is important to make them consciously. Too many good intentions fail because the price of success is not considered when the priority is set. The key here is to consider the price of achieving something important to you and if it's worth it accept the price and pay it. The price of a slimmer, fitter body is probably more time exercising and a change in diet. Recognizing this up front and accepting it frees up mental energy to pursue the goal and makes achieving it much, much easier.

3. Practice Generous Selfishness

When you dedicate time, energy, and focus to your health and well-being, this is both selfish and generous. It's selfish because you aren't necessarily helping others while you are out on your walk or taking extra time to prepare a healthy meal with fresh ingredients. But it's generous when you look at the big picture: Staying healthier lets you be there for others longer, molds you into better shape mentally and physically, usually puts you in a better mode, and maybe even makes you a better provider for you and your family.

4. First Things First

A simple pencil and piece of paper remain your most powerful productivity tools. Keep in mind that the reward for gaining productivity is making time for what's important to you in life – no small task. Starting each day with a list that ties to your goals lets you prioritize and do the first things first. Getting the most important tasks of the day done first (like the morning walk) creates a sense of accomplishment and momentum for the whole day, and it also means that you can't skip them later.

5. Reclaim Your Focus with a Digital Detox

When you take back control of your focus and productivity, you'll find that tasks seem to go faster, you have more concentration, and you get more done instead of spinning your wheels in the service of your devices. (These devices are supposed to be for *your* convenience, by the way. You aren't supposed to drop everything when they beep.) I recommend starting with a full week of total digital detox to regain mental focus. For most people, this will be easier while on a vacation from work. Tell your friends and colleagues you'll see them in a week and sign off. After a few days of adjustment, you will be amazed at the mental clarity that emerges. After the detox, schedule one day a week "off" from all digital interaction, including social, Internet, email, and even (gasp) TV. Finally, regain your daily mental focus by checking email and social media just three to four times per day at scheduled intervals and close it when not checking to avoid alerts and constant distractions from streaming feeds.

6. Don't Pretend to Multi-Task

The theory that multi-tasking let's us "get more done" has been solidly debunked by science. Use this insight to improve your productivity by focusing on one thing at a time, doing it well and to completion, then moving on. Single-tasking (or "being productive," as it was called before computers) is an incredibly powerful self-management tool that is only recently being rediscovered. Turn off the TV, radio, and live feed while you've got important thought work to do and get more done in record time. As a bonus, you'll have more time to really enjoy the entertainment once the work is done.

EATING WELL

"Your body is the direct result of what you eat
and what you don't eat."

—*Gloria Swanson*

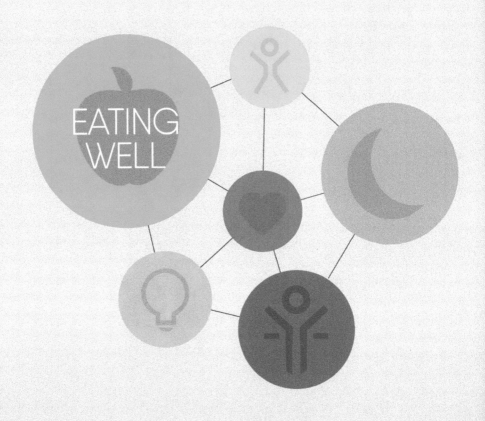

EATING WELL

E ver since reading the book *Sugar Blues* over 30 years ago and experiencing for myself the dramatic difference simple dietary changes can make, I've made the link between nutrition and health my obsessive focus. Food is by far the biggest single chemical we put into our bodies each day—literally the building block of our bodies. Our diet has a surprisingly strong influence on how we look, feel, and act each day, in addition to influencing our long-term health. Every day, science is validating the link between health and diet. Improving nutrition is, in my view, the single most important field of endeavor for improving the human condition.

When Did Eating Well Get So Complicated?

Which is harder to figure out: how to do your taxes or how to eat a healthy diet? In a 2012 survey, the International Food Information Council Foundation asked 1,000 Americans that question—and *52% said it was harder to figure out how to eat healthy.*[13]

Eating is about the most natural thing we do, after breathing. How have people come to see it as being so complicated? Surely, science and common sense must have some absolute lessons about how to eat to keep our bodies nourished and at a healthy weight.

For our Paleolithic ancestors, the decision of what foods to eat was simple—they ate the best foods they could find or catch. The diet changed according to local flora and fauna and time of year. It appears that our ancestors ate a varied diet of fruits, nuts, berries grains, legumes, roots, and other plant matter augmented with fish and game. Their diet was most likely high in variety (because no single food was overly plentiful) and nutrients (because foods were fresh and unprocessed) and low in simple starches and sugars and total calories. They naturally sought out foods that were sweet or fat because these rare pleasures indicated a high-caloric content that would fuel their active, scarcity-driven lives. Even during the past several thousand years leading up to the modern era, constant, abundant, calorie-dense food has been an unattainable dream for most people through recorded history.

It's only over the past century that we have achieved this dream of making cheap, abundant, great-tasting food available to billions of people. In the process, we have created a massive industry of growing, processing, and distributing food to whole countries. The Standard American Diet (SAD) is built around the types of foods that are economical and profitable to produce and distribute more than what is healthy for us to eat. Although scarcity and starvation have, thankfully, been eliminated for many of us, our biological drive to eat foods that are sweet and fat has not gone away, and food producers have exploited this by making manufactured food more appealing by loading them with sweeteners, fats, salt, and other additives (typically, with the cheapest ingredients available to minimize cost and to maximize profitability).

The SAD is now comprised of 70% processed food, on average. The consumption of this fat-, sugar-, and additive-laden food promotes obesity and, as a result, most Americans are unsatisfied with their weight and diet. The same survey that found people were confused about how to eat a healthy diet also found that 55% of Americans are actively trying to lose weight, compared to only 22% who are seeking to remain at the same weight.

With over half of Americans actively trying to lose weight, not only is food production a big business, but weight loss is as well. (Americans spend more than $60 billion a year on weight loss products![14]) With so much money on the table, no wonder people are confused about diet and weight loss. While big food companies are offering us fat-, sugar-, and additive-filled foods, health gurus are decrying the unhealthiness of our diets—but often pitching a faddish, new diet in its place. After all, very little money can be made in common sense, "eat your veggies and get some exercise" kinds of advice.

The good news is that *plenty* of scientific research exists about what constitutes a healthy diet, and none of it is particularly faddish. Of course, many of the diet plans get certain parts of the equation right, or the fads wouldn't have caught on. But many also tend to go overboard. In this chapter, we'll look at the SAD and some alternative ways of eating to see what works and what doesn't. Then I'll give you my prescription for ten things you can do every day to simplify a healthy diet and start Eating Well.

It's Called SAD for a Reason

To have some context on what we *should* be eating, let's start with what we, as a country, *are* eating. As noted previously, it's SAD. It's characterized by lots of corn-fed meat, simple carbohydrates like white flour and potatoes, fried foods, chemical additives, saturated and hydrogenated fats, and lots of refined sugars and additives. It's also extremely high in processed and prepackaged foods. For a mental image of the SAD, picture a super-sized, fast-food hamburger with fries and a soda, plus a candy bar for dessert.

These foods are easy to make in centralized factories and ship out to stores, mini-marts, shopping malls, and fast-food restaurants. It's pre-prepared and packaged for quick and convenient reheating in a microwave or cooking in a deep fryer. The meat comes from densely concentrated feedlots where animals are fed subsidized corn and soybean feeds rather than their natural diets. The animals are given heavy doses of antibiotics to fatten them up and stave off diseases that result from these cramped, unnatural farming conditions. It is loaded with engineered food additives meant to make it shelf-stable and appealing to eat. This standard food is very convenient to ship, store, and quickly serve to suit the modern American lifestyle very well.

In broad strokes, the SAD is 50% carbohydrates, 35% fat, and 15% protein.[15] The carbohydrates are mostly simple sugars and refined flours. The fats are primarily saturated fat—much of it from cooking oils retained from deep-frying. The SAD is equally characterized by what it mostly *doesn't* include, such as enough fiber and complex carbohydrates, vegetables and other plant-based foods, fish, dietary fiber, fermented foods, and healthy fats. As we look at diet patterns, it's extremely important to consider not only what they include, but also what they leave out.

Here are some striking facts about the SAD:
- Each year, the average American eats over 15 pounds of sweeteners and 74 pounds of added fat.[16] (Here, "added fat" means a fat not present in the food but added during processing. So the fat that naturally occurs in beef is not considered added fat, but the oil it is cooked in is.)
- Less than a third of Americans (32.5%) eat two or more servings of fruits each day, and only about a quarter (26.3%) eat three or more servings of vegetables. A serving is a half-cup of vegetables or a piece of fruit the size of a baseball.[17]
- Americans average 12-18 grams of fiber per day,[18] [19] compared to the 20-35 grams per day that experts believe are necessary for good health.[20]
- On average, Americans get 11.3% of their daily calories from fast food,[21] spending a total of $110 billion dollars per year on fast food.
- One in four Americans eats fast food *every day*.[22]
- Food researcher and bestselling author Michael Pollan says that 20% of American food intake is eaten in the car.[23]

Does this diet promote health? Is it eating well? One way to assess how healthy a diet is—or isn't – is to look at the health statistics of large populations that adopt a certain diet.

THE STANDARD AMERICAN DIET

IN ONE S.A.D. YEAR	
Food	Pounds
Dairy	630
Sugar & HFCS	140
Wheat Flour	134
Red Meat	110
Fats & Oils	85
Poultry	73
French Fries	29
Artificial Sweeteners	24
Ice Cream	24
Pizza	23

70%
PROCESSED
FOOD

When I write about a diet, I am generally not talking about "going on a diet," as in a proscribed set of food rules designed to help a person lose weight, like the Atkins Diet or Weight Watchers Diet. Instead, I'm referring to the broad dietary habits of a population. The Standard American Diet (SAD) is the foods that most Americans eat today across the broad population. Many Americans have dietary patterns that are far different than the SAD, but by and large, statistically, this is how people in this country eat. Similarly, the Mediterranean Diet is a pattern of eating based on how people in several countries around the Mediterranean Sea ate at the time the phenomenon was first studied. These countries all had their own national cuisines and dietary habits, but a lot of commonality was found between them that researchers could look at as a diet.

SAD Results: Diet and Health in America

Since the SAD is the prevailing diet in the United States of America (U.S.), it's pretty easy to assess how well it affects our health. Moreover, the U.S. is one of the world's richest and most modern nations and spends more than any other country on health care. In broad terms, we can really focus on U.S. health statistics as being strongly correlated to our prevailing diet. So what do the statistics say about American health? With all our wealth and spending on health care, we should be doing pretty well, right?

In 2013 the National Research Council and Institute of Medicine released a 378-page report on the health statistics of 17 developed nations—*and the U.S. came out dead last in almost all measures of health.*[24]

In life expectancy, U.S. men rank 17th (out of 17), and U.S. women rank 16th. The study found that the low life expectancies disproportionately came from early deaths. Americans have one of the lowest likelihoods of surviving to age 50. We have the second-highest death rates from coronary heart disease (CHD) and also from lung disease.

These are not new phenomena—they have been emerging for the past 30 years. Now, some of these deaths can be attributed to factors not directly related to diet, such as the large numbers of gun deaths in the U.S. that are not seen in any other developed nations. But even if these are removed from consideration, the U.S. does just as badly in these statistics. To the surprise of many of the researchers, these early deaths seem to cut across socio-economic lines. The study's authors note:

"The U.S. health disadvantage cannot be fully explained by the health disparities that exist among people who are uninsured or poor, as important as these issues are. Several studies are now suggesting that even advantaged Americans—those who are white, insured, college-educated, or upper income—are in worse health than similar individuals in other countries."
25

Particularly vexing is *that the U.S. ranked third worst in mortality from nutritional deficiencies, even though we consume more calories per capita than any other nation in the world.* In fact, over 60% of adults ages 20-74 are overweight, with more than a third being obese.[26] Ironically, most Americans are also malnourished—lacking one or more essential nutrients.

Looking at the health outcomes of this type of diet, it *clearly* is not promoting good health. *As a nation, we are both overfed and undernourished—and we are living shorter lives because of this.* If we are going to judge the SAD by how healthy it is making us, then we can only see it as a dismal failure.

There is a second way of assessing a diet, and that is to look at the components that it includes and omits and consider the various implications each of these have on our health.

Refined carbohydrates (also known as simple carbs or processed carbs)
If a food is white, there's an excellent chance that it is a refined carbohydrate, since nature doesn't really make many white foods (save cauliflower). Examples are sugars and white flours. Potatoes are a little more complex, being vegetables, but the way that Americans most often consume them—peeled and fried or mashed— turns them into simple carbs.

Refined carbohydrates have had the nutrients stripped from them, primarily to reduce spoilage, but also to provide a more refined, whiter, supposedly better-tasting product. This allows these foods to be shelf-stable for a long time, but it also means that there is little nutritional value to the food, other than pure calories. These simple, refined carbohydrates break down quickly and trigger the body to release insulin to manage the resulting glucose spike. Once this high dose of insulin has done its job, you start to feel hungry again, due to the blood sugar crash. As this pattern continues, the body eventually becomes less sensitive to the insulin, and this insulin insensitivity is a precursor to diabetes.

Refined carbohydrates—in large proportion—contribute to obesity and diabetes. The SAD consists of roughly 35% refined carbs. These empty calories are a major reason why Americans suffer from both obesity and malnourishment.

Fats make up 35% of the calories in the SAD[27], and most of these are saturated fats. A lot of research shows that saturated fats aren't as bad as we used to think[28], especially the more natural forms like you might find in virgin coconut oil or pasture-raised beef. However, the saturated fats in the SAD tend to come from feedlot beef and worse, deep-fried foods. Heating oils to high temperatures for frying can change the chemical makeup to produce toxic compounds.

The worst possible form of fat—the stuff that absolutely does harm to our bodies—is partially hydrogenated fat and its by-product. Hydrogenation is the process of adding hydrogen atoms to fats and oils. It makes unsaturated fats, like canola seed oil, semi-solid and stable at room temperature, like a saturated fat. As an example, many of us grew up eating foods made with and fried in Crisco shortening, because in those days, everyone was sure that it was a healthier alternative to lard (it's not).

Hydrogenated fats are hard at room temperature, like saturated fat. They make a flakey crust, like lard. And they are much more shelf-stable than liquid oils, which can go rancid. So they are conducive to creating foods in factories and shipping them all around the country for sale in little plastic wrappers. Oh, and they're cheaper to produce. All in all, hydrogenated fats are the factory food jackpot. Unfortunately, they have been shown to cause coronary heart disease (CHD) due to something called *trans* fats.[29] The process of hydrogenating fats creates *trans* fats (named for the type of chemical bond created in the molecule). *Trans* fats raise low-density lipoprotein (LDL) cholesterol and lower high-density lipoprotein (HDL) cholesterol. The Food and Drug Administration (FDA) issued a distinction that *trans* fats are not "generally recognized as safe," and they must now be labeled in all foods.[30]

Feed Lot-Raised Meat

We all need protein, and meat is one of nature's richest sources. Meat also contains many important B vitamins and minerals. Many people worry about the fat content in meat, especially red meat. However, natural meats include a variety of fats, including saturated and monounsaturated. A meta-analysis of several studies has shown that saturated fat from meat consumption does not adversely increase the incidence of coronary heart or vascular diseases.[31] That said, much of the factory-raised meat consumed in the U.S. is fed with corn and soybean meals that reduce the level of beneficial omega-3 fatty acids, compared to more natural feed, such as in grass-fed beef. Grass-fed beef has roughly half the fat of grain-fed beef of the same breed. A greater percentage of its saturated fat content is stearic acid, which has been shown not to adversely affect serum cholesterol as compared to the fats in grain-fed beef, which *do* negatively affect cholesterol levels.[32] Grass-fed beef is also higher in omega-3 fatty acids, beta carotene (a fat-soluble antioxidant), and conjugated linoleic acid (CLA), a nutrient from pasture-raised ruminant animals like cattle that has been shown to lower body fat.

While unprocessed meats have been shown not to contribute to CHD, the opposite is true of processed meats. A very large survey study at Harvard University with data from 20 studies and over a million subjects concluded that, "Consumption of processed meats, but not red meats, is associated with higher incidence of CHD and diabetes."[33] Meats preserved with nitrites (bacon, hot dogs, sausages, salami) have also been shown to form carcinogenic compounds, and they are listed as Group 1 carcinogens by the World Health Organization – the same category as smoking tobacco.[34] This is because processed meat consumption has been associated with a higher incidence of colorectal cancer. So if you eat meat, the best bet is to stick to unprocessed, lean cuts of grass-fed animals.

Another health concern with meat consumption is that when the fats on meat are charred—as typically happens in barbecuing, deep-frying, broiling, and smoking— carcinogenic polycyclic hydrocarbon compounds form. This is the main reason I avoid all beef in my own diet.

So, unprocessed meat is probably fine in moderation, but processed, preserved, and charred meats are the hallmarks of the SAD. These are not consumed in moderation. In 2012, Americans ate an average of 180 pounds of red meat and poultry. This is 53 pounds (42%) more than in in the 1950s.[35] So while meat itself may be healthy in small doses, that's not what most Americans are eating.

Preservatives and Additives
When you make foods out of highly refined ingredients, you need to add a lot back into it to make it tasty. That's what the packaged food industry does with its products. Between sugar, salt, monosodium glutamate (MSG), and other natural and artificial flavorings, our food is loaded with additives. Preservatives such as butylated hydroxyanisole (BHA), butylated hydroxytoluene (BHT), and benzoates help make food survive cross-country transportation and stay fresh on store shelves. But once in the body, they kill our native beneficial gut probiotics. These additives have each individually passed FDA reviews, but as a cocktail they are very concerning. No matter how you look at these additives, they are adding a lot of chemistry to our food. And whether or not they are damaging by themselves, there's no denying that the reason they are put into food is because the food is not nutritious, flavorful, or fresh enough to stand without them.

Antibiotics
Healthy cattle, chickens, pigs, and turkeys are regularly fed antibiotics and antimicrobials because it helps them put on weight faster and with less feed. According to the World Health Organization, three times more antibiotics (by

volume) are sold for animal uses than human use.[36] This overuse of antibiotics is rapidly creating antibiotic-resistant bacteria.

In 2001, *The New England Journal of Medicine* published a study that found that 20 percent of supermarket ground meats (beef, chicken, turkey, and pork) contained *Salmonella* bacteria and of that, 84 percent was resistant to at least one antibiotic.[37] Another study found that people became infected with *Salmonella* resistant to treatment with ciprofloxacin hydrochloride after eating pork.[38]

The Food and Drug Administration studied penicillin- and tetracycline-based animal food additives between 2001 and 2010, and the results were only released through a Freedom of Information Act request and subsequent litigation from the nonprofit group the Natural Resources Defense Council. In 2014, *The New York Times* reported that the released documents showed that of 30 common antibiotic feed additives, *18 posed a high risk of exposing antibiotic-resistant bacteria through food.*[39]

The exposure to these antibiotic-resistant bacteria from our food is troubling in itself, but antibiotics in meat also concerns me because it is reflective of the unhealthy conditions where the animals are raised and the goal of putting on as much weight as possible at the cheapest cost, which is the core of factory meat production. Animals raised in a healthier manner, such as pasture-raised animals, don't have the need for so many antibiotics. And because they eat their natural foods, their meat is much healthier for us to eat.

Low Amounts of Fiber

Dietary fiber is indigestible carbohydrate that comes in two forms: soluble and insoluble. Soluble fiber, found in oats, barley, legumes, citrus, apples, and some vegetables, dissolves in water to form a gel. It lowers cholesterol levels and moderates blood sugar. Insoluble fiber mostly keeps things moving through your gut at a good pace. All fiber slows down digestion so that even sugary foods spike blood sugar less. Fiber also fills you up so that you feel less hungry, even after consuming fewer calories.

Fiber is extremely important for intestinal health. Many types of indigestible fiber are actually eaten by prebiotics, our beneficial intestinal flora from which the bacteria create short-chain fatty acids required by the colon and liver. Different bacteria feed on different forms of fiber, and it appears that people who eat a wider variety of fruits and vegetables have more diverse populations of beneficial bacteria. (This is covered more fully in Pillar Five: Hosting Well.) The average American eating the SAD gets about half the recommended amount of dietary fiber.

Vegetables contain fiber, vitamins, minerals, and numerous phytonutrient compounds that we have only recently begun to recognize. Human beings evolved to eat a lot of vegetable matter. And while there may be some extreme populations that get by without vegetables, by and large, the more veggies that are included in a diet, the healthier its people tend to be.

Vegetables are extremely important for our health. The USDA Food Pyramid recommends eating 3-5 servings of vegetables per day and 2-4 servings of fruit. Frankly, this is probably on the low end, and we should be eating a lot more vegetables. In 2009, however, only about a quarter ate three or more servings, according to figures from the Centers for Disease Control and Prevention (CDC), and both of these percentages had *fallen* since 2000.[40]

But even these numbers are too optimistic. About 10-13% of the U.S. population identifies themselves as vegan or vegetarian, so we can assume that these folks are *definitely* getting several servings of vegetables each day.[41] [42] Take these hard-core vegetable consumers out of the equation, and it appears that only about a fifth of non-vegetarian Americans eat two or more servings of vegetables per day and even fewer eat three servings.

Few Healthy Fats

Fats can be saturated or unsaturated. Generally speaking, unsaturated fats[1] are considered healthier than saturated fats. Understanding fats is not quite as simple as we once believed, however. We know that partially hydrogenated fats are unhealthy, but beyond that things are not always instantly clear, largely because fat has been such a villain in the public perception. For example, virgin coconut oil, while high in saturated fat, raises the good HDL cholesterol, thus improving the HDL/LDL ratio. It increases LDL too, but much less than HDL, and it's the ratio of the two that is most important. Saturated fats high in stearic acid (chocolate, beef, butter) have been found to be associated with lower LDL levels and seen as not having a negative effect on cholesterol levels. However, in general, saturated fats do tend to raise serum cholesterol levels, particularly LDL.

Unsaturated fats, however, can be quite healthy, particularly the omega-3 fats from fish and seafood, as well as walnuts and flax seeds. Polyunsaturated fats, such as olive oil, avocados, sunflower seeds, and cottonseed oils, seem to have heart-protective qualities, especially when they replace saturated fats. The SAD is low in these healthy fats, except for corn and soy oils. However, corn and soy oils lose their health benefits when used for frying because the high heat changes the nature of the oil molecules.

Fermented foods like yogurt, sauerkraut, kimchi, pickled olives, and cheeses contain beneficial bacteria that can help replenish our natural microflora. While the health benefits of yogurt and other fermented foods have been long known, only now are researchers beginning to appreciate the full importance of our microflora. (See Pillar Five: Hosting Well.)

Diets rich in fermented foods seem to have a host of health benefits. A study published in 2013 in the *Journal of Medicinal Food* tracked 100 young men who ate an identical diet except for the amount of kimchi they consumed (none; approx. 1 ounce; approx. 8 ounces). After one week, the kimchi-eating groups had lower total cholesterol, LDL cholesterol, and fasting blood glucose than the control group—and those who ate the most kimchi had bigger drops.[43] This result is similar to other studies that have found improved cholesterol and blood glucose from oral probiotics (the isolated bacteria from fermented foods). Unfortunately, kimchi and other fermented foods do not make up a large part of the SAD.

Low Amounts of Fresh Fish

Many of the world's healthiest diets include a lot of fish. Fish has quality protein and healthy fats, particularly omega-3 fatty acids, which reduce CHD through their anti-inflammatory and other properties. Fish and seafood are also seen as beneficial because they typically replace red meat in a meal, which often has a less desirable fat profile (i.e., more saturated fat). The average American eats just over 14 pounds of fish and 82 pounds of chicken per year. For comparison, the average Japanese eats 120 pounds of fish per year, and the average Spaniard eats 96 pounds of fish per year.

Overall Calories in the SAD

Beyond looking at the components of the SAD, we need to consider the amounts consumed. Americans have the highest average caloric intake in the world. Why is that? Well, one clear factor is the amount of refined sugars and other carbohydrates we consume. These give us a double-whammy: they set up a cycle of blood sugar spikes and crashes that keep sending us back for more simple carbohydrates. Since these calories are largely devoid of nutritional value, our bodies continue to crave real nutrients like vitamins, minerals, and healthy fats, so we eat more.

Excessive serving sizes that come with the SAD are a big culprit here. As part of my work, I travel to Europe several times a year. One thing you notice right away in Europe is that the people are a lot thinner. In fact, less than 30% of Europeans are overweight or obese, compared to over 68% of Americans. One of the secrets is in portion size. European portions seem to be about half the size of American portions. But you feel just as good an hour after dinner and better the next morning. Try "Eurosize" portions – cut your normal serving in half and see the difference.

If the SAD is a good example of how not to eat, what should we eat instead? Let's look at two diets that are very popular today because of their claims of improving health. We can assess their pros and cons and see if we can learn some lessons about how to eat for our best health in the real world we live in today.

The Paleo Diet

The Paleo Diet craze began with Walter L. Voegtlin's book *The Stone Age Diet,* published in 1975.[44] However, the trend really hit its stride in the past decade, ever since Loren Cordain published *The Paleo Diet* in 2002.[45] It is extremely popular at the moment, and many bestselling books advocate some version of it.

The basic tenets of the Paleo Diet are that our bodies evolved over millions of years to eat a varied diet of meats, fruits, and vegetables like that of our Paleolithic ancestors, and we are unable to properly process agricultural products like grains, legumes, and dairy and particularly food additives, like sugars and other chemicals.

What does a Paleo Diet look like? It is characterized by lots of meat, fish, green vegetables, nuts, and healthy fats. It does not include any dairy, grains, legumes, processed foods, or alcohol. Imagine a big surf and turf barbecue with a salad, some broccoli, and maybe some berries for dessert but no cheese, milk, beer, or wine to go with it.

One of the reasons why the Paleo Diet is popular is that many elements of it are *gigantic improvements* over the SAD. Right off the bat, it eliminates sugary drinks and refined starches, which gets rid of several pounds of added fat each year and helps prevent the blood sugar roller-coaster ride that so many Americans suffer from on the SAD. The vegetables help ensure better nutrition. And while a lot of meat is consumed with the Paleo Diet (often more than the SAD, since some Paleo proponents suggest two-thirds meat to one-third plant-based foods) it is in the unprocessed variety—which has a much healthier protein and fat profile than feedlot meat. So in many important respects the Paleo Diet is a big upgrade on the SAD.

Can we study any populations to assess how healthy the Paleo Diet is? Unfortunately, it's pretty impossible to find any Paleolithic people still running around to study. However, a study of the people of Kitava in the Melanesian Islands actually helped spur the Paleo Diet craze when it found that the people of Kitava ate a diet uninfluenced by Western diets—something close to the Paleo Diet that was to follow—and suffered no reported heart disease or stroke whatsoever.[46]

While it does make some instant improvements over the SAD, the Paleo Diet also has some problems. First, we need to understand that at the moment, it is an

THE PALEO DIET

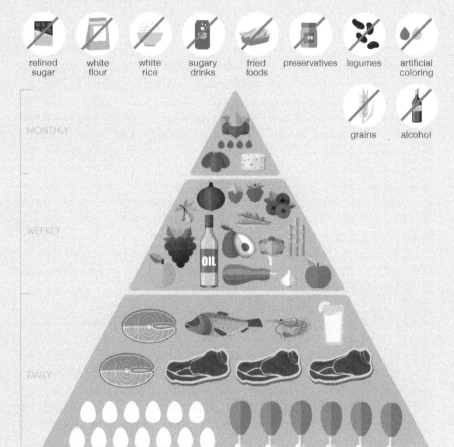

refined sugar · white flour · white rice · sugary drinks · fried foods · preservatives · legumes · artificial coloring

grains · alcohol

MONTHLY

WEEKLY

OIL

DAILY

invented diet rather than some real mode of eating that exists anywhere in the modern world. The "Paleo Diet" of these proponents is not the diet of the Kitava people, which consists mainly of coconuts, fruit, and fish. It's a diet based on a lot of assumptions, and it has not yet been measured in any broad populations.

The Paleo Diet begins with the presumption that the 10,000 years since humans adopted agriculture have not been enough time for human evolution to adapt to agricultural products like grains and dairy. However, is this really true? Five thousand years ago, human beings only drank milk during breastfeeding. Therefore, the gene for producing lactase—the enzyme that breaks down lactose—switched off after infancy. However, in Northern Europe, a genetic mutation called lactase persistence arose and spread through the population. It allowed people who possessed it to access a new and important food source—dairy products.[47] This was so important that it spread through most of Europe in a relatively short time. A similar but independent mutation occurred among West African pastoral populations, also enabling them to drink milk. It spread among these populations so that over 90% of some of these populations also possess it.[48] This mutation is now common enough in people of European descent that we actually see it as the *norm*[2] and call the previous normal, non-mutated condition "lactose intolerance." It's clear, then, that humans can evolve and pass along new genes rather quickly when they open up an important new food source.

Humans adopted agriculture around 10,000 years ago. Certainly some would have lacked the proper enzymes to take advantage of these new crops. However, very quickly (in evolutionary scales) those who could process grains, legumes, and other agricultural produce would have prospered under these new food sources and quickly outpaced the productivity in terms of passing on their genes versus those who could not digest these foods. Within a few generations, the progeny of grain-eaters would be very well suited to digesting these grains. The idea that 10,000 years is not long enough to adapt is a misleading argument: it sounds good until you really examine it. New archeological evidence is also showing that pre-agricultural humans still ate grains and legumes.[49] They just didn't *grow* them yet. After all, why would people choose to farm foods that they didn't actually eat?

The Paleo Diet[3] makes a lot of concessions to the modern world. For example, it allows coconut oil, which is very healthy for eating and cooking. But where was a caveman supposed to get his hands on any coconuts? Moreover, the meats and vegetables that the Paleo Diet allows are just as much products of human agricultural selection as those it omits. A Paleolithic person would no more recognize the Brussels sprouts allowed by the program than the green beans that are not. Further, the very high amounts of meat that the program advocates are troubling for me, based on what the scientific observation has revealed about meat consumption since the days of the caveman.

I admire a lot of individual elements of the Paleo Diet. However, because of the emphasis on meat over plant-based foods, and because it rather arbitrarily omits all grains, legumes, alcohol, and dairy, as well as many fruits and vegetables. I don't believe it is the ideal eating system, despite some important advantages over the SAD. We are modern humans who retain a lot of the dietary machinery of our ancestors from the past 100,000 years. However, we also live in a modern world and must choose the best options from the full cornucopia of modern foodstuffs available to us. There's no real benefit to pretending that we have not changed in the past 10,000 years of agriculture when all signs say differently. If I had to choose between only the SAD or the Paleo Diet, I'd take Paleo hands down (though I'd go heavy on the veggies). Fortunately, we don't have to make this choice. Science shows us better options are available.

The Mediterranean Diet

The Mediterranean Diet is probably the healthiest way of eating in the world. Like the Paleo Diet, it offers a better alternative to the SAD. But in most respects, it is very, very different from the Paleo. The first difference is where the diet originated, in the cultures living around the Mediterranean Sea. The connection between the traditional diet of these cultures and lower cardiovascular disease was first noted by Scotsman Dr. Samuel Black in 1819. In 1958 a study of diet and health began in the U.S., Japan, Finland, the Netherlands, Italy, Yugoslavia, and Greece to look at men's diets versus their incidence of heart disease. Known as the "Seven Countries Study", it has been going on for over 50 years.[50] One of the great observations this study made was that men from the countries bordering the Mediterranean Sea had far less incidence of heart disease than men from the U.S. and Northern Europe, even controlling for other factors. And these Mediterranean men consumed high levels of dietary fat, which at the time was believed to be a strong factor in heart and vascular disease. This was called the "Mediterranean Miracle," and it forced scientists to look deeper into the diets of these countries to understand why they could eat so much fat and still have a far lower incidence of the killer disease.

The Mediterranean Diet as we know it is characterized as consuming large amounts of olive oil, legumes, whole grains, fruits and vegetables, and fish; moderate amounts of dairy as cheese and yogurt; moderate alcohol (mostly wine); and low amounts of meat. It is a bit of a mixture of the generally common, healthful dietary habits of many groups living around the Mediterranean. These groups were mostly Crete, other parts of Greece, Southern Italy, and Spain in the 1960s, where the phenomenon was initially studied. A typical meal would look like a number of different dishes in small portions, like Spanish tapas—mostly plant-based foods, lots of olive oil, seafood, a little meat and a glass of wine, with cheese and fruit for dessert. This meal would generally be eaten slowly (by American standards) with family and friends.

THE MEDITERRANEAN DIET

refined
sugar

fried
foods

sugary
drinks

preservatives

artificial
coloring

moderate
alcohol

MONTHLY

WEEKLY

DAILY

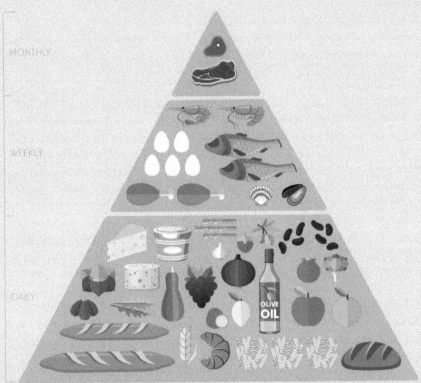

We could examine numerous real-world populations that incorporate this type of diet. In fact, that is how it first drew attention. So what do we learn from studying these groups? Well, in addition to the cardiovascular benefits shown in the Seven Countries Study and others, a recent study published in *The New England Journal of Medicine* in 2013 found the astounding fact that **the Mediterranean Diet cut the chances of heart attack, stroke, and death from heart disease by 30 percent among 7,447 Spaniards ages 55-80 who had significant risks factors for heart disease, including smoking, diabetes, and being overweight.**[51] This reduction is comparable to taking a statin drug. The subjects ate a Mediterranean Diet including a lot of fish, legumes, olive oil, vegetables, and nuts instead of a more typical Western Pattern Diet (another name for the SAD). The results were so conclusive that the study was actually ended early—after about five years—because it was considered unethical to continue to force the control group to go on. Cutting the risk of a cardiovascular event that could lead to death by 30 percent is a truly astounding amount from diet alone and gives a lot of substantiation to the benefits of the Mediterranean Diet.

Researchers have found numerous other medical benefits to the diet. A 2008 study by the *British Medical Journal* found that the Mediterranean Diet provides substantial protection against type 2 diabetes.[52] A different 2008 meta-study by the *British Medical Journal* found that strictly following the Mediterranean Diet reduced the risk of dying from cardiovascular disease by 9% and cancer by 6%,[4] as well as reducing the incidence of Parkinson's and Alzheimer's diseases by 13%.[53] In other words, the Mediterranean Diet has a lot of real-world research showing it to be strongly protective against a wide variety of health threats.

Because the Mediterranean Diet is based on the way real people in developed nations eat today, it's actually quite easy to incorporate into our diets. I think this is very important. If you want to adopt a Mediterranean-style diet, you can easily find these foods in grocery stores and restaurants, so you can still participate in a normal social experience and stick to this time-tested way of eating. This is far more important that many people realize. Adopting a very odd, hard-to-achieve diet like the strict Paleo Diet sets a person up for failure and frustration and insulates them from normal social experiences, which are also a key part of living well.

The Mediterranean Diet is, in many ways, an inverse of the Paleo Diet. It has low amounts of meat but very high amounts of fiber and antioxidant rich plant-based foods, including all fruits and vegetables (preferably in a wide variety) plus (mostly whole-) grains and legumes. It also includes alcohol, mostly in the form of wine. Yet some important commonalities are in both diets. They both include healthy fats, seeds, and nuts, while they limit or eliminate refined sugars and flours.

Research into the Mediterranean Diet continues as scientists look to understand the components that have the most impact. A few key players have emerged: healthy fats from olive oil and nuts; a high variety and proportion of vegetables, legumes, and grains; high fish and seafood consumption and low red meat consumption; moderate wine and alcohol consumption; fermented foods; and largely slower, more social eating.

Supplement Support

Having spent my entire professional life at the intersection of nutrition and health while living in the real world, I know that it's tough to maintain this perfect eating program every single day. Working with my team of scientists and nutritionists, I sort out the fake from the real in the world of nutrition for a living and have been exposed to very promising research on the link between certain supplements and health. Put simply, even if you are eating well, a few specific supplements can support your health in ways that even nine servings of fruits and vegetables cannot. That's why I routinely take a few supplements that I suggest you add to support the Eating Well Pillar. The following supplements are the ones I take every day, in addition to Eating Well, because they have been rigorously studied and have significant health benefits.

Purified Fish Oil

I take 1,000 mg of a highly purified omega-3 fish oil supplement, because I can't always get enough seafood. I would rather get a little too much omega-3 than risk not getting enough. Unfortunately, enough mercury is in the ocean food chain now that it can concentrate in fish oils, so only take fish oil that has been purified using the "supercritical CO_2" method. This process uses very cold carbon dioxide gas and no chemical solvents to extract the omega-3s from the fish oil. It leaves behind all mercury and other impurities.

Mediterranean Plant Nutrients

All the research I've done on the Mediterranean Diet has convinced me that vital components are in that way of eating that are important to get every day. Now, emerging scientific research is confirming that resveratrol, lycopene, lutein, and olive polyphenols may have an enormous positive effect on health. These natural compounds are called phytonutrients (or plant nutrients), since resveratrol is in grapes, lycopene is in tomatoes, lutein is in green leafy vegetables, and olive polyphenols – especially hydroxytyrosol – are in olives. I take specific forms of these nutrients invented by some of the research doctors I work with in my nutrition practice. These are clinically demonstrated to absorb better than generic supplements.

I take 100 mg of resveratrol, 7 mg of lycopene, and 10 mg of lutein in this form every day, along with 100 mg of olive polyphenols. In addition, I take the lycopene and lutein at different times of day, because they compete for absorption in the body.

You have probably heard about the benefits of red wine. These benefits are thought to come from resveratrol, a powerful polyphenol and anti-fungal chemical found in the skin of grapes and also found in red wine, in small amounts. Resveratrol is one of the most exciting nutrients around because of its power as an antioxidant and its role in slowing the rate of cellular aging. Harvard-educated researchers Dr. Christoph Westphal and Dr. David Sinclair conducted genetic research on resveratrol and call it the fountain of youth.[54] But not all resveratrol is created equally.

Resveratrol is made by the grape plant to fend off fungal infection, so the amount varies widely by growing region and by levels of pesticides used on the grapes Pesticide use means the plant does not need to make any resveratrol. So not much resveratrol is in each glass of red wine (less than 1 mg for wine not grown organically). In addition, the ill effects of excessive alcohol use would far outweigh the benefits of resveratrol alone. Resveratrol in the "trans" form – the form the body can use – can be harvested in very high concentrations from other natural plant sources. This provides the resveratrol content equivalent of over 100 glasses of red wine in a concentrated supplement.

We know that oxidative stress and chronic inflammation are characteristics of many diseases, such as cardiovascular diseases, insulin resistance, auto-immune diseases like rheumatoid arthritis, and Alzheimer's disease. A new study published in the *Journal of Clinical Endocrinology and Metabolism*[55] examined the result of a trans-resveratrol-containing plant extract on oxidative stress and inflammation, by measuring its suppressive effect on reactive oxygen species (ROS) generation and a range of inflammatory mediators. The study states, "Resveratrol may reduce oxidative stress and inflammation through increased expression of anti-inflammatory cytokines, and a reduction in pro-inflammatory molecules." The promise of resveratrol has attracted hundreds of millions of dollars in research.

In the body, resveratrol is known to protect cells from oxidative damage and may play a role in activating pro-longevity sirtuin genes. That's one reason resveratrol is a popular beauty-inside supplement. But standard resveratrol supplements have very low bioavailability (the amount of a given dose of a substance that is actually available for your body to use) and thus probably don't do much. Working out of Cambridge, England, cardiologist and researcher Dr. Ivan Petyaev invented a process that significantly enhances resveratrol's bioavailability in supplement form, and that's the one I take. His patented process starts with natural resveratrol in its trans form. In combination with the antioxidant carotenoid lycopene, it builds natural micelle structures around resveratrol molecules to enrobe them in lipid coating at the microscopic level for significantly enhanced absorption. In clinical tests, this form of resveratrol was shown to have superior bioavailability when compared to regular resveratrol supplements.[56] Further, this resveratrol-lycopene combination was shown in a published clinical trial[57] to help heal skin lesions on the feet of patients with diabetes. This is proof positive of its ability to protect cells from damage.

While the results of the study are promising, many researchers believe there is much more to the Mediterranean diet than just resveratrol.

Lycopene Limits LDL

We know that Mediterranean people also feast on the freshest fruits and vegetables, such as locally grown, ripe tomatoes. Unlike the store-bought variety we find here, the traditional Mediterranean diet calls for vibrant red, vine-ripened tomatoes. The carotenoid that gives tomatoes their distinctive color when ripe is called lycopene, and it is another powerful antioxidant. In the body, lycopene is known to support cardiovascular health, to protect skin from sun-induced aging, and to limit LDL cholesterol oxidation. In fact, a landmark 1995 study of 47,894 men conducted by Harvard University found that eating ten or more servings a week of tomato products was associated with a reduced risk of prostate cancer by as much as 34 percent.[58] In another recently published study, men who had the highest amount of lycopene in their body fat were more than three times less likely to suffer a heart attack as those with the least amount of lycopene in their body fat. Lycopene in body fat is an indicator of lycopene content in the diet.[59]

Lutein for Healthy Macula

Lutein is another carotenoid and is a powerful natural antioxidant found in green leafy vegetables, an important part of the Mediterranean diet. In the body, lutein is known to concentrate in the macula of the eye to support eye health and also in the skin to provide antioxidant protection and to support healthy skin.

I work with computers much of the day (and sometimes much of the night), and the blue light that screens emit can damage the macula over time. So I take 10 mg of lutein with another carotenoid called zeaxanthin that occurs naturally with lutein in food sources. This is delivered in micelle form developed by Dr. Petyaev, so I'm confident about absorption. Since macular degeneration is the leading cause of blindness in the U.S., a lutein/zeaxanthin supplement is a good idea for anyone with a family history of macular degeneration.

Olive Antioxidants

One of the newer supplements I've recently added to my regimen is an antioxidant from olives, a staple in the Mediterranean Diet. Researchers have found that the key antioxidant in olives and olive oil is a compound called hydroxytyrosol. Olive oil hydroxytyrosol was the marker compound used in the largest-scale study ever published on the subject (in the prestigious New England Journal of Medicine). This study included more than 7,400 people in Spain and found that the Mediterranean

Diet group had a 30% lower incidence of cardiovascular events, stroke, and death than the standard diet.[60] Because of the implications for public health, the study was stopped early so the information could be released to the public.

After reviewing the research on the Mediterranean Paradox in detail, genetic scientist Dr. Roberto Crea also had doubts that wine alone was fully responsible for its protective benefits. Recently "retired" at a young age following the hugely successful public offering of his employer Genentech, he bought a large olive grove in northern California because it reminded him of his native Italy. Dr. Crea began tinkering and investigating. He tested the product of his organic olive groves and discovered the most potent antioxidant from olives was *not* in the oil, but in the water being squeezed out of the olives during processing. Dr. Crea discovered that while polyphenols are present in extracted olive oil, olive oil water contains even higher concentrations of these polyphenols.[61]

Could the key to the Mediterranean Paradox be in the olive oil water? This component, hydroxytyrosol, had been wasted in the modern method of processing olives, which dramatically reduced the antioxidant value.

Dr. Crea developed and patented a two-step process to utilize olive water rich in antioxidant polyphenols. First, the pits are removed from the pulp of the olives. Then pitless pulp is crushed and washed with water to obtain a paste of olive oil and vegetation water. Finally, the water is separated and processed with citric acid to stabilize the ingredient, retaining the highest antioxidant activity.

A recent article published in *Pharmacological Research* states, "An olive extract rich in hydroxytyrosol may protect neurons in the brain from the normal deterioration associated with aging."[62] The study concurs with Dr. Crea's findings that hydroxytyrosol is the main antioxidant compound in olives and is believed to play a major role in the many health benefits attributed to olive oil, such as cardiovascular health. This research also states, "Results showed that the olive oil compound (hydroxytyrosol) reduced the cell damaging effects of the oxidative and nitrosative stress in a dose-dependent manner, with higher doses providing increased protection." Researchers believe this may reduce chronic inflammation, which accompanies conditions like heart disease, diabetes, arthritis, and Alzheimer's.

Based on my familiarity with Dr. Crea's research, I take 100 mg of his hydroxytyrosol-rich olive extract every day. In the body, hydroxytyrosol is active as an antioxidant in both fat- and water-soluble structures of the body and may play a role in activating pro-longevity sirtuin genes. In clinical tests, Dr. Crea's olive juice extract was shown to have 300 times the antioxidant activity of extra-virgin olive oil without the fats or calories. Independent laboratory analyses have demonstrated that hydroxytyrosol is one of the most potent natural antioxidants yet discovered.

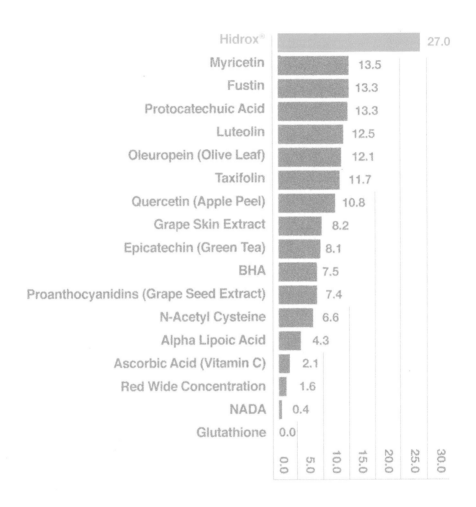

	ORAC Value
Hidrox®	27.0
Myricetin	13.5
Fustin	13.3
Protocatechuic Acid	13.3
Luteolin	12.5
Oleuropein (Olive Leaf)	12.1
Taxifolin	11.7
Quercetin (Apple Peel)	10.8
Grape Skin Extract	8.2
Epicatechin (Green Tea)	8.1
BHA	7.5
Proanthocyanidins (Grape Seed Extract)	7.4
N-Acetyl Cysteine	6.6
Alpha Lipoic Acid	4.3
Ascorbic Acid (Vitamin C)	2.1
Red Wide Concentration	1.6
NADA	0.4
Glutathione	0.0

The rigorous study mentioned earlier was published in *The New England Journal of Medicine* in 2013. It involved 7,447 participants in Spain over a five-year period. This study found that those who followed the Mediterranean Diet, supplemented with either extra-virgin olive oil or nuts, experienced "a relative risk reduction of approximately 30%, among high-risk persons who were initially free of cardiovascular disease. These results support the benefits of the Mediterranean Diet for cardiovascular risk reduction."[63] Hydroxytyrosol was the key marker researchers used to measure compliance with the Mediterranean Diet, and long-term adherence provided these remarkable results.

PRESCRIPTION №2

1. Cut the white stuff, especially sugary drinks

2. Swap healthy fats for fried foods

3. Eat protein and fiber at every meal

4. Maximize variety, especially with veggies

5. Moderate alcohol consumption

6. Rest your digestive system

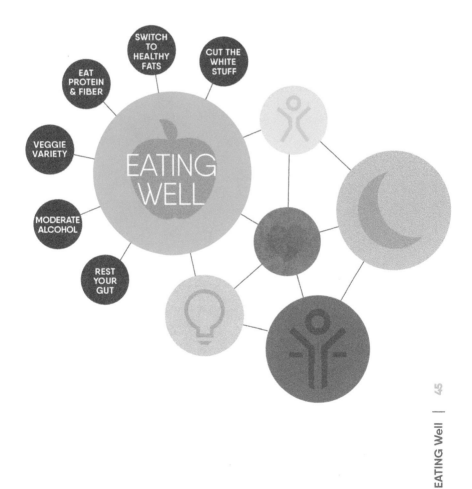

THE LIVING WELL DIET™

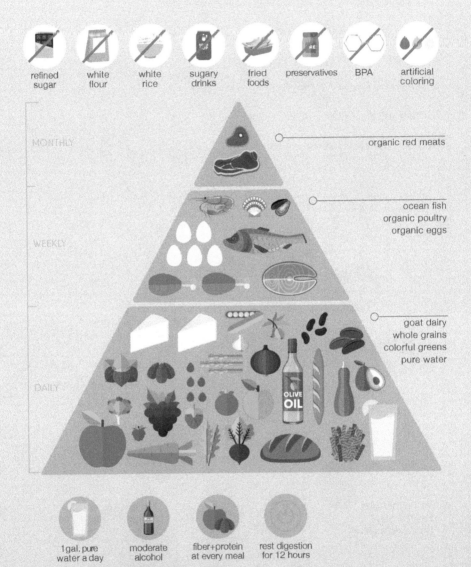

refined
sugar

white
flour

white
rice

sugary
drinks

fried
foods

preservatives

BPA

artificial
coloring

MONTHLY

organic red meats

WEEKLY

ocean fish
organic poultry
organic eggs

DAILY

goat dairy
whole grains
colorful greens
pure water

OLIVE
OIL

1 gal. pure
water a day

moderate
alcohol

fiber+protein
at every meal

rest digestion
for 12 hours

The Living Well Diet™

We've looked at three ways of eating—the Standard American Diet, the Paleo Diet, and the Mediterranean Diet – and examined data about how they work (or don't) for our health. There are many other diets that we could examine in depth here: Ketogenic diets (75% fat, 20% meat, 5% carbs, so not very sustainable or practical), the French Paradox[5] (rich in antioxidants and probiotics) and the Okinawa Diet (voluntary calorie restriction), for example. Instead, I'm going to combine many of the lessons I've come away with after studying dozens of these real-world dietary models. Each has something to teach, because each shows the long-term results of a certain national cuisine and allows us to compare what is eaten (and not eaten) with broad health outcomes. I've translated the science for you here and have created, what I believe to be, a better eating plan for a healthier life. This is The Living Well Diet.

I believe that if you are constantly worrying about exactly how many grams of this nutrient or that you are consuming, then you probably aren't living life to the fullest. You probably aren't going to stick to any highly restrictive diet long-term, either. Rather than being on a diet, I believe it is much healthier to simply have a diet that helps you live well.

The "85% Rule"

My goal with these "prescriptions" is to give you simple, achievable actions that you can do without constantly adding up food points or calories and finding a way to eat well for the rest of your life. I also believe the "85% rule" applies as the right percentage of the time to stay strictly disciplined and have found that to be the right ratio for making health-positive changes permanent. To stay on a healthy eating plan for your lifetime, you need to enjoy it, and you need to give yourself some flexibility. About 15% of the time works for me. You can suffer through a month or two of an exception-free weight-loss diet program that you don't really enjoy, but that's won't work when creating a lifelong eating plan.

Eating well is meant to be enjoyable and achievable over a lifetime. After all, how many "diets" encourage you to make sure to have a drink or two every day? However, some parts of the plan may be more difficult for some people to adopt right away. If some part of the plan is particularly challenging for you, then by all means, adopt the other elements and work toward incorporating the missing element(s) as you can. While there is a synergistic effect of adopting all elements of the plan, it's far better to do most of the steps than none of them.

Don't worry about complying with 100% of the steps 100% of the time. Stressing out about your diet is *not* living well. I've found that 85% is about right. In fact, the stress could be more counterproductive to your health than the occasional "cheat meal."

On a personal note, this is the way I have eaten for years and have stayed within 5-10 pounds of my high school graduation weight. So my recommendations are based on both research and direct experience. In fact, I have seen marked improvements in my health, well-being, and enjoyment of life. But I don't follow the plan 100% all the time. If it's someone's birthday, I have a small slice of cake—sugar, refined flour, and all. This is a lifetime plan. I'm not going to go my whole lifetime and stay on any eating plan perfectly, and neither are you. I am for adhering to the program at least 85%.

From looking at the longitudinal studies, my educated guess is that the thousands of people following the successful eating programs researched for years and years probably had an extra drink or a dessert as a treat once in a while, too, without skewing the results. For me, sticking to the program at least 85% gives me the results I need. I would encourage you to follow the program as closely as you can, but accept that in a lifelong eating plan, there will be some slip ups and missed objectives. Just move on and try to do better the next day. The goal of The Living Well Diet™ is to help you live life to the fullest.

1. Cut the White Stuff, Especially Sugary Drinks

Nature doesn't provide many white foods like sugar and flour, and cutting simple sugars and carbohydrates is the best place to start Eating Well. In all my research, I could not find any generally healthy populations that consume large portions of their daily calories from refined flours, sugars, and high fructose corn syrup (HFCS) calories, either through foods or beverages. (In fact, even the Inuit diet of 50-75% fat calories and 35-40% protein seems to be far healthier.[64]) So cutting sweet beverages, sweeteners, and refined flours is probably your fastest step for a healthy diet and a healthy weight. The easiest way to do that is to stop buying them and to stop drinking them.

Liquid calories were never a common occurrence for our ancestors. As a result, our bodies don't have a good mechanism for handling these, especially when they contain newer, highly processed sugars like HFCS. These liquid calorie bombs spike our insulin, but because they don't come with any fiber to slow down digestion—as whole fruit would—our bodies don't kick in the normal satisfaction hormones that tell us when we are full when we drink sugars.

Numerous studies have shown that when we eat a 100-calorie slice of bread, our bodies reduce our hunger response and caloric intake for the rest of the day (especially if it's whole wheat bread with fiber, vitamins, and healthy fats). However, that same 100-calories from a soda or glass of apple juice does not reduce our hunger response. [65] [66] So it's an *extra* 100 calories over what you would normally eat as opposed to the bread, which will count against your body's daily set point of calories it seeks.

How big a problem are these liquid calories? On average, each American drank 44.7 gallons of bottled soda in 2010, according to *Advertising Age* magazine.[67] If a person drank 44.7 gallons of regular soda in a year, that would equal 66,752 additional empty calories. There's no nutritional value to these calories, and as the studies show, they don't satisfy your hunger. They are pure extra energy that is typically converted to body fat. At 3,500 calories per pound of body fat, that is *19 pounds of additional fat each year* that an average person could gain just from consuming sugary sodas. Now, some of these sodas may have sugar-free artificial sweeteners, but those are fraught with their own health issues.

And the sodas don't even tell the whole story, because the same article reported that each year, Americans also average 18.5 gallons of packaged coffee, 10.3 gallons of tea, and 11.5 gallons of fruit beverages. These are pre-packaged beverages, not the coffee or tea people make for themselves or order at a coffee shop. The coffee and tea are by and large sweetened. And while fruit juices may include some nutritional value, they are not the same as whole fruit, with its fiber and real nutrition. These sugary fruit beverages also spike our blood sugar without producing satiety (the feeling of fullness that tells us to stop eating), so they are also *extra* calories. That's another 40.3 gallons of sweetened beverages and perhaps another 40,000 empty calories, or 11 pounds of additional body fat each year. *That's a combined 20-30 fat pounds worth of excess calories that the average American would put on (or have to work off through exercise) through drinking sugary beverages every year.*
Now, most people manage to burn off a large percentage of that 20-30 pounds of fat per year, but often not all of it. However, managing this annual fat means that a person is not burning off the fat they've already accumulated.

These consumption facts are shocking but explain the obvious. Why are so many Americans overweight or obese? Because we are consuming 20-30 pounds of body fat-producing calories that we put on each year through consuming additional—empty—calories from sugary beverages. If you could make only one improvement on the SAD that would have the greatest impact, this is it: cut out all sugary beverages and save those calories for something nourishing.

Fortunately, this is a pretty simple change to make. People tend to drink soda and other sugary drinks out of habit. Habits can be hard to break, to be sure—however, substitutions exist. Plain water is a terrific substitute for any soda. If you find you miss the carbonation, then carbonated water is a good replacement (and fun to do with a SodaStream machine). If you are used to the caffeine, then freshly made, unsweetened coffee or tea (or naturally sweetened with a plant-based sweetener like Stevia) will deliver that buzz, along with a healthy dose of beneficial nutrients. It only takes a week or two to retrain your taste buds to appreciate unsweetened coffee and tea. The one substitution I don't recommend is diet soda. While you will cut the calories, these artificial sweeteners are, in many ways, just as unhealthy as sugary drinks.

Diet beverages have actually been shown to contribute to weight gain. They create Insulin releases that can give a person a sugar crash without having eaten any real sugar. This sets up diet soda drinkers to eat more calories than they would otherwise.[68] In a 2008 study, rats fed artificial sweeteners were found to gain more weight than those fed sugary diets.[69] So it's true that diet soda actually makes you fat.

Fruit juices are also mostly empty calories. Most fruit juices really only wear the cloak of healthy food. In actuality, their real nutrients are lost in processing and shipping, and they only have vitamins because they have been chemically added back. You are far better off eating a piece of fruit. *In fact, please do.* You will get the full benefit of the fiber and nutrients, plus your body will account for these calories and reduce your hunger. Real fruit also produces a much lower blood sugar spike than packaged juice.

While you're eliminating empty calories from beverages, it's wise to also cut out as much HFCS from other foods too. Consuming HFCS makes the body resistant to leptin, the hormone that makes us feel full.[70] That's one reason why foods with HFCS may contribute to obesity, by making the eater never feel full or satisfied. So consuming foods with HFCS may make you eat a lot more during a meal than you would otherwise, because you just don't feel full.

A study released in 2014 by the *Journal of the American Medical Association – Internal Medicine* looked at the health effects of sugar. It found that sugar not only makes people fat, it is making them sick as well. This study found that overall, Americans consume about 15 percent of their calories from added sugars. Sugars that occur naturally in fruit are not considered added sugar. About 10 percent of adults get 25 percent or more of their calories from added sugar. The risk of dying from heart disease for people getting this much sugar was 38 percent higher than those who consumed only 7 percent of their calories from added sugar.[71]

The study found that people who drink one sugar-sweetened beverage per day have a 29 percent higher chance of dying from heart disease than someone who drinks one per week. The risk of cardiovascular disease rose exponentially as the amount of sugar in the diet increased.

One of the simplest steps you can take to improve your health is to eliminate all sodas, whether sweetened with sugar, corn syrup, or artificial sweeteners. None of these are doing your body any good. Replace these with water or unsweetened coffee or tea. Cut out processed fruit juice and energy drinks while you're at it.

These are faux health foods that don't do you any good. Check labels for HFCS and corn syrup and eliminate or reduce foods containing it.

This one step could save you from having to deal with pounds of added body fat each year from empty calories. You might feel a bit run down for a day or two as your body adjusts to healthier fuel from food, not corn sugar, so it's best to drop the sodas over a weekend. By Monday, you will feel a different, more even, and less erratic energy. Your body will avoid blood sugar spikes and crashes, and you will have better clarity and focus.

After the first two weeks, you will retrain your brain to seek out and recognize the flavors of the actual foods and beverages you are enjoying, rather than always looking for sweetness. That's why I recommend dropping *all* added sweeteners. If you can't bear the thought of that, then use small amounts of natural reb-A extract from the leaf of the stevia plant, which is natural-sourced and calorie-free.

The SAD is loaded with "white stuff" like sugar and flour in the form of processed foods. They fit in very well with our always-on-the-go lifestyle, and they're usually inexpensive and always so convenient. They're tempting, too, thanks to chemical additives designed to trigger the pleasure centers in our brains. Many processed foods contain chemicals that tap into the same brain receptors as marijuana.[72] But these processed foods are unhealthy. They set us up for spikes and crashes in our blood sugar and generally undo all the good we are accomplishing with the rest of our dietary habits.

In America, we are simply desensitized to packaged, processed foods. But that is not the historical norm. If a food is in an individual plastic wrapper, if every piece looks essentially like every other piece, or if you can really only tell what the heck you're eating by reading the package it came in, then you are probably eating an overly processed food. And all the nutrition has likely been stripped from it before you ever bought it.

Don't settle for nutrition-stripped foods. I can't see any evidence of healthy populations who eat a lot of processed food. Why should you eat something that doesn't give you any nutrition? Cut out these empty calories in favor of food that will benefit you more than simply filling up your belly for a few minutes until your next sugar crash.

I would love to tell you to cut these foods out altogether. You'd certainly be healthier for it. However, I'm not sure that's realistic in today's society. Instead, I recommend that you limit your intake. Be conscious of when you are eating processed foods. The more packaging and the less you can identify by sight the components of a food, the more processed it is. So much of the SAD is processed food that we are completely used to it now. So I'm suggesting that you become aware of it again and limit these obviously processed foods to one per day.

2. Swap Healthy Fats for Fried Foods

In 2000, Americans averaged 64 pounds of added cooking fat per year, up from about 31 pounds per year in the 1950s. This is out of a total of 85 pounds of fats and oils we eat each year. *Our use of added cooking fat has more than doubled.* This is the fat used to cook and flavor food and does not include the fat content of the food itself. Those 64 pounds of cooking fats add up to over 250,000 calories per year.

Unlike the added calories and body fat gained from sugary drinks, our bodies do account for the extra calories from dietary fats. In fact, fats make us feel very full. Many fats are quite beneficial and even necessary to our health. However, the fats from fried food, especially as these fats are used in the SAD, are not healthy for a few important reasons.

Frying changes the composition of oil. Many oils that have been touted as healthy, such as canola, soy, and corn oil, quickly degrade in high-heat frying and create toxic compounds that lead to hardening of the arteries and other health concerns. By and large, food in the American diet is fried in saturated or hydrogenated oils, or it is cooked in an otherwise healthy polyunsaturated oil that becomes unhealthy due to high-heat frying.

Additionally, in most American cuisine, frying involves coating the food in a flour batter that absorbs more grease and combines it with simple carbohydrates for a double-hit of empty calories. Many people order chicken sandwiches at fast food restaurants, thinking they are a healthier option than a hamburger, without realizing that the fried chicken patties have twice as many calories.

Cutting out fried foods could save the average American well over 100,000 calories per year, or 300-plus excess calories per day. It also eliminates many toxic burned oil compounds and hydrogenated oils, which both adversely affect cholesterol levels.

Certain fats are important for our health, but not the kind we get from fried foods like French fries, potato chips, and fried chicken. These frying fats are typically saturated or hydrogenated. And even when unsaturated fats are used, the high-heat frying alters their chemical makeup to create toxic substances. Remove deep-fried food from your diet altogether. If you are eating the SAD now, this step alone can take off ten pounds or more in the first few months of your new way of eating.

Fats have been demonized across the board, but some good fats also exist. Over the past 30 years, Americans have continuously reduced their fat intake, but over the same period, our bodies have gotten a lot fatter. When we reduce dietary fat, we tend to replace it with carbohydrates, particularly sugar, since we need to add a lot of flavor to make up for the missing fat. Eating healthy fats, on the other hand, offers a high degree of satiety – the feeling of fullness. It fills you up quickly and makes you feel satisfied so you don't binge later. If you want to gain some weight, go eat a lot of "reduced fat" products.

Remarkably, many regions have people who are healthy despite their high dietary fat intake. The Mediterranean Diet is one example. The French Paradox, with all its cheeses and *foie gras,* is another. Somehow these regions and others have high dietary fat, often even saturated fat like the French, Inuit, or Kitava people. Yet they show far less coronary disease than Americans with similar fat intake. A number of factors come into play, including exercise, but the specific types of fats consumed are a primary reason for this difference.

The Mediterranean Diet has a high intake of healthy fats, particularly from olive oil and nuts. Olive oil is loaded with monounsaturated fats, and it is the primary fat used for both cooking and flavoring food, in the same way that we would put butter on bread. Some people believe that the olive oil's main contribution is that it replaces less healthful saturated fats. But this seems unlikely, as these fats are proving to be less harmful than once thought. More likely, the powerful antioxidant components in the olives are actively benefitting health.

Olive oil has one of nature's most potent antioxidants, hydroxytyrosol, and numerous phytonutrient compounds. Even more of this natural protective substance is in whole olives. An 11-year study in Spain found that, unlike cooking oils used in the SAD, food cooked in olive oil do not contribute to heart disease.[73] These fats also come with a healthy amount of phytonutrients, unlike many fats in the SAD.

The Mediterranean Diet includes other healthy fats as well, including omega-3 fatty acids from fish and other seafood plus seeds and nuts. A recent five-year study followed participants who were already eating a Mediterranean Diet and found that those who added nuts to their diet were 30 percent less likely to have a major cardiovascular event, and 49 percent less likely to have a stroke.[74] So, more healthy fats seem to be even more protective.

Other populations with good cardiovascular health also eat a lot of healthy fats (and get plenty of exercise). The Inuit get enormous amounts of saturated fat from their diet, but they also burn huge amounts of energy keeping warm. More importantly, the fats are from natural seafood, which, while loaded with natural saturated fats, is also rich in omega-3 fatty acids. And the Kitavu people are getting an enormous amount of saturated fat from coconuts. This fat is a fairly unique type of saturated fat that our bodies seem to be able to process very well. In fact, lauric acid, the type of saturated fat that makes up most of coconut oil contains medium-chain triglycerides that are metabolized directly by the liver for quick energy, unlike most fats. And our bodies convert lauric acid to monolaurin, a compound that is only found in one other food source; breast milk.

So when you look at the various "Paradox" and "Miracle" diets, you discover that they often contain high levels of fats, but they are specific beneficial fats like polyunsaturated olive oil and other nut oils, omega-3 fats, and virgin coconut oil. By including these in your diet, you will feel satisfied with how much you eat, and you will eat fewer carbohydrates. The carbs you do eat will also digest and release their sugar more slowly, due to the fat in your stomach.

Eating the right types of fats will help you feel full so you can stop eating. They'll also improve your cholesterol levels and balance. What are the right types? Extra virgin olive oil is the granddaddy of healthy oils. Omega-3 oils from fish and seafood are also extremely beneficial. Plant-based versions of omega-3 oils are not quite as powerful as the versions from seafood but still well worth including in your diet. Nuts and seeds offer rich sources of these healthy fats as well. Virgin coconut oil is an excellent fat that our bodies process differently than most other saturated fat. All of these oils in their minimally-processed forms are better than butter, which is almost pure milk fat.

How much of these fats can you eat? Again, I want to set guidelines for healthy eating, not specific daily targets to hit. But you may find it shocking, given the villain role that fat is usually cast in, that I recommend that you eat as much healthy fat from these sources as you like—*as long as you are also doing all the other recommendations in Living Well, exercising daily, and getting eight hours of sleep per night.*

When our body chemistry isn't out of whack due to chronic sleep debt or wild swings in blood sugar, our bodies do a great job in limiting the amount of fats we consume. At some point, too much dietary fat makes us feel really full, so we stop on our own. The hard part with omega-3s is getting enough, not too much. Recently some researchers have found that there may be some negatives in extreme doses of omega-3 fatty acids, but they concede that these amounts are far beyond what a person could get with a normal diet *plus* typical supplements.

I recommend cutting out fried foods altogether and getting at least one to two grams of omega-3 fats per day. One serving of salmon or anchovies covers this.

Most healthy diets include some protein at every meal, and it's not always as obvious as a meat dish. Many cuisines have paired staple grains and legumes. Typically, neither one contains all the essential amino acids, or protein building blocks, on their own, but in conjunction they do. This is why you constantly see beans and grains combined in traditional cuisines around the world: red beans and rice, corn and pinto beans, rice and soy, wheat and lentils. These grain and legume combinations create complete proteins without any meat.

Eating protein slows the absorption of sugars and starches, which reduces blood sugar spikes and crashes that encourage binge eating. Protein is slow to digest and requires more energy to consume than either carbohydrates or fats, and it provides the building blocks for cell regeneration. A dieting myth says you should separate carbohydrate meals from protein meals, but there's no strong scientific evidence that this is beneficial. It's better to eat a balanced diet and to include some protein at every meal.

Meat is a very easy way to get protein. If you favor meats that are pasture-raised, you won't have to trim the fat away. They will be naturally leaner, and the fats will tend to have a healthier lipid profile due to the animal's natural diet. Cheese and dairy are good sources. A glass of milk has about eight grams of protein, so a great way to turn an all-carb snack into something more complete and healthier is to add a glass of cow's milk or one of the many milk alternatives rapidly taking market share (almond milk is my favorite). The fats and protein will slow the absorption of the refined carbohydrates and smooth out the blood sugar spike and crash.

Seafood also makes for great protein options. When eating seafood, however, it's best to eat from low on the food chain to avoid accumulated mercury. Large predatory fish like tuna and swordfish accumulate all the mercury from the fish they eat and pass this highly toxic metal on to us when we eat them. Smaller fish like anchovies, sardines, and even wild salmon carry less toxic mercury. Shellfish can also be great and delicious protein sources with low mercury levels. Shrimp, oysters, clams, and mussels are among the lowest in methylmercury content.

Eggs are a remarkable protein source. Somehow, eggs got an undeserved reputation as being unhealthy. It's probably due to the saturated fats in the yolks. However, egg yolks are packed with vitamins and hard-to-get nutrients like biotin that, in moderation, are well worth any fat they may contain. Two eggs have 15 grams of complete protein, or all essential amino acids, in a form that is very easy for your body to use.

Eating protein gives our bodies the raw materials it needs to build various compounds we require to live and grow. I don't think there's any need to constantly monitor your protein intake. As long as you are eating a protein-rich food, or a combination like rice and lentils, at every meal, you will easily reach the goal of 50 grams of protein per day. For example, a cup of milk and a slice of whole wheat toast has more than 10 grams of protein. So does two eggs or a serving of yogurt. Even a small serving of meat or seafood will give you ample protein for that meal. As long as you are consciously including a complete protein source, you will easily meet this prescription.

What you want to avoid is having low protein meals or snacks, such as a meal of toast and jam or pasta and tomato sauce. Add some milk or yogurt to that toast or toss in some shrimp or cannellini beans with the pasta to add protein easily and deliciously.

I recommend that you get at least 50 grams of protein daily and eat protein with each meal.

Fiber slows down initial digestion and prevents blood sugar spikes. It also keeps food moving through our digestive systems so that our processed food doesn't hang around in our bodies as long. This is one of the reasons why high dietary fiber intake is associated with a reduced risk for colorectal cancers. It literally pushes things out of our guts faster so that harmful substances don't form or stick around long enough to do damage. Fiber also lowers our blood cholesterol levels and feeds our beneficial flora that help keep us healthy. (More on this in Pillar Five: Hosting Well.) And on top of all that, it makes you feel full, so smaller meals feel satisfying, and you can reduce some of the high-caloric intake that Americans have come to accept as normal.

The healthiest diets seem to incorporate high levels of dietary fiber from vegetables, legumes, and grains. Due to its high amount of plant-based foods, whole grains, and legumes, the Mediterranean Diet includes a high amount of fiber. One study in Spain found an average fiber intake of almost 30 grams per day and postulated that this may be a key component of the Mediterranean Miracle. The American Dietetic Association recommends 20-35 grams per day, and the average American gets about 12 grams per day.

Thankfully, fiber is pretty simple. Yes, two kinds exist, soluble and insoluble. but they occur in reasonable proportions in a number of foods. As an easy reference, an apple has about six grams of fiber. When you're getting the proper amount of fiber from several different kinds of foods, you won't have to worry about the ratio of soluble to insoluble, because you'll be getting plenty overall.

A higher level of fiber is going to fill you up faster, so you won't have to worry too much about the actual number of calories you're getting. Honestly, what's worse than counting calories and being hungry? It's so much better to get full on high-fiber foods so that you don't suffer with hunger, which always drives you to binge in the end and leaves you an empty stomach to shove lots of sugary calories into. Fiber is the key to digestive happiness. One of my favorite sources of fiber is chia seeds, which have about 11 grams of fiber per ounce, along with omega-3 fatty acids, protein, and antioxidants. I mix a couple of tablespoons with yogurt for my first meal of the day and have more than a third of my fiber requirement covered.

While The Living Well Diet is not a plan that requires a lot of monitoring and tracking of calories, fats, and sugars, fiber intake is a good parameter to track, at least for the first three to four weeks. Fiber is shown clearly on every food label. By adding up your total fiber each day, you will get a sense for what adequate fiber intake looks like and feels like. Most people are poor judges of how much fiber they're eating, so writing it down for a while is a good way to build your awareness.

Tracking your intake throughout the day also helps you recognize when you're not getting enough so that you can eat a fiber-rich dinner. Here's a hint: one big bowl of bean or lentil soup can easily cover half your daily fiber requirements. Of course, it's best to spread this out across your meals rather than to try to get it all at once. After you've done this for a few weeks, you'll have a sense of what adequate fiber intake looks like and feels like, and it will come more naturally to you.

I recommend that you get 30 grams of fiber per day from a variety of plant-based foods.

4. Maximize Variety, Especially with Veggies

The Mediterranean Diet is high in vegetables and other plant-based foods, and these occur in a wide variety. People end up getting a lot of different phytonutrients from the plants. In addition to the well-known nutrients like Vitamins C and D, our bodies can benefit from hundreds, maybe thousands, of plant nutrients. Science is still discovering these and learning what roles they play in our health. Many don't even have names yet. But by eating a wide variety of fruits, vegetables, legumes, nuts, and grains, the people of the Mediterranean countries are able to benefit from having these in their diet, even without knowing what they are. Variety staves off nutritional deficiencies and promotes good health.

The great success of human beings is that we can live in a lot of places and survive on a lot of types of food. As people living in a modern world, we should embrace this. Get a wide variety of fruits and vegetables. Eating a variety of foods helps ensure that we get all the micronutrients our bodies need.

From a health and sustainability standpoint, I admire the local food movement, the idea of trying to mostly eat foods raised within a reasonable radius of where you live. I think trying to incorporate this into your food buying is both admirable and healthy, since foods with less time to market tend to retain more nutrients. However, we should also acknowledge that we live in a modern food distribution environment where we have the amazing privilege of buying bananas, apples, kale, and leeks in the same section of the supermarket almost any day of the year. This is available to us for the first time in history on such a broad scale, so let's take advantage of it and eat this fantastic abundance we have to choose from.

Even with all of these food choices from around the world, Americans get most of their calories from ten crops or food sources: corn, wheat, rice, potatoes, tomatoes, chicken, beef, pork, eggs, and milk/dairy. Many populations that have good health and long lives tend to eat from a variety of different foods. This is one of the benefits of living in a modern society. There are plenty of health shortcomings to modern life, so let's take the good where we can. Enjoy a wide variety of foods, and you don't have to spend time worrying about whether you got all the nutrients you need, because you naturally will.

It's common to get into a rut and have the same breakfast every day and the same few options for lunches and dinners. If you expand your food choices, you'll enjoy food more because of it, and you'll get a wider variety of nutrients. You'll also have a better chance to avoid getting too much of any toxins that might be in a certain type of food.

Consciously eat for variety. Try to have four identifiable foods on your plate for any given meal. Then aim for a different set of foods at each meal. By the end of the day, you will have likely consumed more than a dozen different foodstuffs. That's great variety for a given day. If you can carry this variety to the following day, so you're not repeating foods, then you are really starting to get a broad source of meats, seafoods, fruits, vegetables, and legumes for a diverse diet rich in nutrients.

Vegetables are extremely important players in good health. The people in most nations who enjoy long, healthy lives seem to eat plant-based diets with plenty of vegetables. So that's my recommendation for you as well. Fill your plate with vegetables. Make those the centerpiece of the meal instead of the meat course.

The cornerstone of a SAD meal seems to be meat. Ask a friend what he had for dinner, and he's likely to respond with steak, pork chops, or chicken. In the U.S., the meat is often the meal. This is not true everywhere. In many Asian countries, people think of a meal as rice with some side dishes to accompany it. In fact, in Japan, the word for "meal" is literally "cooked rice." I'm going to encourage you to rethink dinners. Instead of being centered around the protein, center meals around the vegetables. The protein may very well be a legume. Traditional Indian and Korean cuisines are constructed in this way, as are many others, and these populations enjoy good health as a result.

So fill up on a variety of vegetables. You will feel full, get a variety of different nutrients, enjoy lots of great tastes, get plenty of fiber, and probably save some money over meat-centric meals. This approach ensures that you get good nutrition and never leave the table feeling hungry. It sounds like a lot, but it isn't hard to do. Vegetables tend to be very easy to prepare. A big mixed salad gives you several servings of vegetables. Just add some olive oil and vinegar as a dressing. Put a small piece of meat or fish on top, and you've got a complete meal. You can steam or roast more than one kind of vegetable at a time for very efficient cooking that doesn't require as much constant care as cooking meat. A baked potato with a couple of side dishes of sautéed vegetables is another great example of filling up on veggies for a satisfying meal.

The idea here is to think about plant-based foods, and specifically vegetables, as the core of your diet. Meat, grains, fruit—those are important players that you'll add to top off your meals. But vegetables are the core. Think this way and things like getting enough fiber and nutrients become almost automatic.

Please pay attention to the "fill up" part of the recommendation. Like most of the recommendations I will make throughout *Living Well*, there is no need to suffer. Fill up! I don't want you walking away from the table feeling hungry but virtuous, because that is *not* living well. That's martyrdom! Plus, you'll end up raiding the stash of dusty Halloween candy at 1 am anyway. So, fill up. Leave the table *full*, satisfied, and really nourished. Fill up on *vegetables* rather than white bread or meat or any of the other nutritionally poor foods that dominate the SAD.

One great way to eat a variety of foods is to buy a variety of foods at the market. When you shop, try to buy a variety of different ingredients and step outside your comfort zone. Avoid loading up on any staple favorites in favor of more variety. When you get home, you'll have the building blocks of meals with great variety.

I recommend having two to three kinds of vegetables per meal. This makes it easy to get six to nine servings of vegetables in a day.

5. Moderate Alcohol Consumption

Moderate wine consumption plays an important role in the Mediterranean Diet. Although it's not completely understood, moderate alcohol intake, or one to three drinks per day, seems to have a protective effect on the cardiovascular system. Wine also has natural phenols and polyphenols, protective compounds from the plants themselves. Resveratrol is the best known of these, but many others exist, and they are still being studied. White wine, for example does not have resveratrol, but does have other components, such as caffeic acid and tyrosol, that seem to have health benefits of their own. Beer has also been shown to be rich in antioxidants and phytonutrients.

If you suffer from cirrhosis or alcoholism or have problems limiting your consumption to a drink or two per day, then by all means, cut alcohol out of your diet. If this does not apply to you, however, the medical literature suggests that drinking one to three alcoholic beverages per day does have health benefits. In fact, recent studies are finding that **people who cut out all alcohol are more likely to die prematurely than people who consume moderate amounts on a regular basis.**[75] The study looked at over 1,800 people aged 55-65 for a 20-year period and was tightly controlled for all important variables. It found that the moderate drinkers (one to three drinks per day in this study) died prematurely at a rate of 41 percent, while 69% of the alcohol abstainers died prematurely, almost double the rate. Even heavy drinkers (four or more drinks per day) had better results than the non-drinkers, with a premature death rate of 60%. While heavy drinking may be statistically healthier than abstaining, it does not lead to a better life. Not all the answers to living well can be found in statistics.

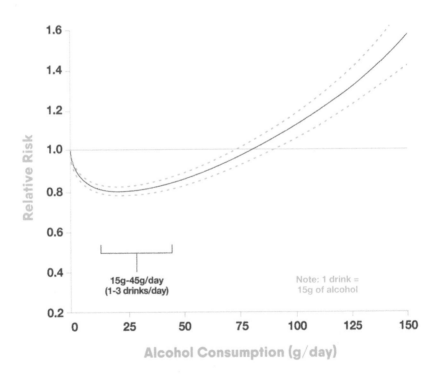

Relative risk of coronary heart disease and alcohol consumption, based on a meta-analysis of 51 published scientific articles. Note that the observed protective effect of alcohol is about one drink/day for women and two to three drinks/day for men. A typical drink contains 15 grams of pure alcohol. The middle line is the result of the meta-analysis, while the upper and lower lines are the confidence intervals.[76]

So it would appear that it isn't just the resveratrol and other polyphenols in the wine that offer health benefits. It is also the alcohol itself.[77] In a 1999 study published in the *International Journal of Epidemiology*, Dr. Hans Hoffmeister calculated that if Europeans stopped drinking beer, there would be a drop in the average life expectancy of two years and a decrease in general happiness.[78] That said, only moderate drinking (one to three drinks per day) seems to have a protective effect. And that protection drops off precipitously at either end of that zone. Also, abstaining, then binge drinking five to six drinks or more per session does not offer cardiovascular protection, even if the overall average falls within the one to three drinks per day range.[79,80]

Diet rules that probably don't apply to you

Americans are fascinated with health and diet news, so startling new studies often make the news. Unfortunately, we also tend to self-diagnose conditions. The supermarket shelves are full of products labeled "low sodium," "lactose free," or "gluten free," and these types of foods have been perceived by many as healthier versions. The fact is, however, only some people actually need to watch their salt intake or avoid lactose or gluten.

It's wonderful that food options are available for people who truly have health conditions that dictate that they must eat this way. However, if you don't have celiac disease, then you don't get any health bonus for avoiding gluten. If you don't have hypertension, there's no great need to moderate your salt intake. If you are not lactose intolerant, then you don't get any bonus points for cutting dairy out of your diet. People worry about damaging their kidneys by eating too much protein, because studies done on people who already suffer from kidney failure show that excessive protein can be a problem *for those people*.[81] If you don't suffer from kidney failure, there's no benefit in limiting protein intake to the levels that are safe for people who do.

I want to encourage you not to self-diagnose medical conditions. If you think you may be sensitive to gluten or lactose, then by all means, go to your doctor and get tested. You may be right, or some other medical condition may exist that only a doctor armed with the proper tests can accurately diagnose. If you don't have a real medical reason to avoid these foods, then don't get caught up in the hype. The food industry is constantly looking for new ways to make its products look healthy, even if they are actually rather nutritionally empty. Don't buy into it and avoid otherwise healthy foods without good reason.

Our ancestors did not have the benefit of refrigerators or pantries stocked to the rafters with easy-to-prepare food. We evolved from people who often waited between meals. Today in America, it seems that the eating never really stops. Many people snack right up until bedtime, wake up for a midnight nosh, and have breakfast minutes after the alarm goes off.

When we eat food, we digest the sugars and starches and convert them into glucose, which we may burn immediately or store in our liver and any muscle cells that have room to hold it (in the form of glycogen) and then in fat. When we stop eating, we continue to digest our food for several hours, especially if we're including protein, fats, and fiber in our meals, which significantly slows digestion. If we eat every four to six hours, we only ever burn the glucose from the foods we just ate. Any excess is stored as fat. But because we eat so often, we rarely dip into that fat to retrieve that stored energy. It takes at least six hours after eating a regular meal before our bodies start accessing fat calories. This is all due to our body's hormone response to food, primarily from insulin production.

I recommend you give yourself at least a 12-hour break from eating each day. This is a lot easier to do than it first sounds, because you'll be asleep for most of that time. The key to making this easy is to finish dinner twelve hours before you would normally eat breakfast and then don't snack before going to bed. If you typically eat breakfast at 8 am, then back up your schedule by ten hours and plan not to eat anything after 8 pm.

A twelve-hour break rests your digestive system so that it is not constantly working. This gives our metabolism a chance to switch from burning the glucose in our food to burning fat for a few hours each day. This is an important process that will help your body shed fat.

Exciting new research supports resting the digestive system all the way from dinner to lunch. This Swedish study was done with people with type 2 diabetes and looked at three diets: a conventional low-fat diet (45-56% carbohydrates), as recommended to most diabetics; a Mediterranean diet with coffee only for breakfast and a bigger lunch (32-35% carbohydrates); and a moderate low-carbohydrate diet (16-24% carbohydrates). Each had the same number of total calories. The results were stunning. The low-fat diet had the worst impact by far on blood sugar levels throughout the day, while the low carb diet showed significantly lower blood sugar and insulin levels all day long. The Mediterranean diet showed lower insulin and blood sugar levels, except for after the big lunch. The implications are intriguing and make me wonder if a combination of a low carb diet, the Mediterranean diet, and intermittent fasting could have a synergistic effect on blood sugar metabolism and fat burning.[82]

Another diet trend that's popular at the moment is called intermittent fasting (IF). Although IF is hotly debated, some people swear by it, and others dislike it for a variety of reasons. This is partly because every person's body chemistry is different, and some people will have a much more positive experience than another with the same amount of fasting. However, it's also because a lot of different fasting plans get lumped under the IF moniker. For example, one eating pattern is to simply extend the daily overnight fasting period, as I recommend here. Some people will extend this daily fast up to 20 hours. This is often accompanied by four hours of eating whatever you want, which I think is counterproductive. This is sometimes called 20-4 IF, for 18 hours of fasting and 6 hours of eating. Similar programs are 18-6 and 16-8.

One version of IF is alternate day fasting, which means eating normally several days a week or every other day, accompanied by fasting all day on the other days. This is sometimes called 5:2 IF for eating normally for five days and fasting for two.

I don't recommend approaches that lead to yo-yo eating, where you feel starved for too long and then rebound and binge on too much food or low quality diets. Remember that calories still count, and we are better off with a Euro-sized than an American-sized portion, even with IF. The studies that do support health benefits from IF are from eating patterns where IF lowers the overall calorie intake.[83] Going without food for many hours is not a good excuse to eat junk.

Yet IF seems to work well for some people, mostly adult men. In men, IF seems to improve insulin sensitivity, while in women, it has no effect or worsens insulin sensitivity, according to one human study of alternate day fasting.[84] Women see less benefit from more extreme IF, and some women report negative effects, including difficulty sleeping, increased stress, and fertility and hormonal problems. These are consistent with results of studies that looked at IF in female rats.[85] Children should not go beyond ten hours without eating, as several studies have shown that it has a negative effect on learning and IQ.[86]

Resting your digestive system for twelve hours is, to me, a minimum number, not a maximum. Adding another hour or more to this period of fasting puts the body into a fat-burning state for longer. Going 13 or even 14 hours is not uncomfortable for many people if they work their way up to it and schedule well. I personally go about 12 hours without eating almost every day by having an early dinner, skipping late-night snacks, and going for a walk first thing in the morning before a mid-morning breakfast, and recommend this as the optimal daily digestive rest for Living Well.

MOVING WELL

"Physical fitness is not only one of the most important keys to a healthy body, it is the basis of dynamic and creative intellectual activity."

—John F. Kennedy

MOVING
WELL

O ur bodies are designed to move every day. Movement helps pump our blood and get our minds working. Regular movement makes us feel better, live longer, and do more. Movement is a virtuous cycle: the more you move, the more you want to move, and the easier moving becomes.

Unfortunately, modern life has taken a toll on our movement. Tens of centuries ago, Paleolithic humans needed to constantly hunt and gather to collect the items they needed to survive. People of the agricultural era also worked long days in fields to secure a living. Today, however, technology has replaced much of the physical work people used to do every day. While that's a great benefit in many ways, it has sapped the movement our bodies need to stay healthy.

Most Americans now work in offices, sitting at computer screens all day after sitting in cars to during the commute to and from home. Once back at home, there's just enough energy to park their tired selves in front of the TV, computer, or iPad to watch videos or play games for hours on end. Our labor-saving devices are saving so much labor for us that we may not be moving as much as we need to ensure our health. How long can this go on before we end up like the hoverchair people in the Pixar movie, WALL-E?

The good news is that this is all easily addressable for free, and the benefits of doing so are very real, starting almost immediately. I've spoken with leading exercise physiologists, scientists, and sports medicine doctors across the country who have made breakthrough discoveries about the positive power of movement for our bodies and minds. One thing I've noticed about these researchers is that they practice what they see working in their research and are all leading active lives. They're not just talking about the power of movement, they're putting what they know into practice. What I'm learning from people all across America and the world, whether scientists or office workers, is that once they start incorporating more movement into their routines, they feel better physically and mentally. Their bodies feel better, they're less tired at the end of their days, and their general stress level is much lower.

This chapter shares some of the surprising things I've learned about movement. They've challenged my thinking about the importance, and even the definition, of exercise and being active, and they've helped me look at the topic in a new way. Let's take a look at what it means to move well and how you can incorporate these lessons into your own life to create positive, lasting changes.

Exercising first thing in the morning has many benefits. Various studies have shown that morning exercise may not only curb appetite[87] and help people sleep better at night, but it may also combat the effects of a high-fat diet[88] and increase fat burning[89]. I've found that moving in the morning really helps eliminate any grogginess and shifts me into gear for the day. And best of all, doing some exercise first thing in the morning means that you can't skip it later when "life gets in the way." It also kicks off a sense of accomplishment that can last all day.

After a night's sleep, our bodies typically need a period of adjustment to fully wake up. Exercise gets everything firing together by getting our blood pumping and our hormones aligned into a daytime state. If you can exercise outside in the sunlight, or my favorite, sunrise, it's even more effective at waking you up.

Imagine how a day might have begun for our ancient ancestors. They woke to the rays of the rising sun flowing through the cave entrance. They push off the animal skins and stumble over to the refrigerator to grab a quick bite of breakfast. Well, okay. That probably never happened. Instantaneous food preparation is a product of the modern era. When early humans woke up, they most likely needed to go out and find some food before they could eat anything.

In the developed world today, food is rarely more than an arm's grasp away from us. Whole industries—fast food, packaged food, vending machines—have sprung up to ensure that no one ever needs to wait a moment for a meal. But that's not what our bodies are used to doing. Growing evidence indicates that going for a few hours between meals might just be beneficial.[83]

Studies have found that exercising before breakfast can help your muscles deal more effectively with blood sugar than exercising after you have eaten, especially for high-fat diets.[90] Walking in the morning may also reduce stress reactivity.[91] Morning exercise starts off your day the right way and takes little time, compared to the boost it gives you.

Beyond feeling better all day, improved self-esteem is a key psychological benefit of regular physical activity. Exercise releases endorphins, brain chemicals that reduce your perception of pain and that just plain make you feel great. This is why we can feel euphoric for hours after a workout, giving us a positive prism to view life's daily challenges when we are not working out.

In Pillar Two: Eating Well, I discussed how extending the fasting period between dinner and breakfast can improve our hormone response to food and give our digestive systems a much-needed break from non-stop food consumption. Many people will wonder whether it makes sense to exercise during this period of fasting. I was curious about this myself. After all, some studies have shown that people get better muscle gain and use more energy by consuming a pre-workout meal compared to exercising in a fasted state.[92] In reviewing this research, it appears that, if you are already a lean bodybuilder or elite athlete looking to pack on the most muscle possible, then you should consume some protein prior to exercise so you don't burn your muscle tissue for fuel. The same applies if you are a child in school, where eating before school has shown to improve academic performance.[93] However, for most people looking to lose weight, exercising before eating has been shown to be more effective at promoting fat loss than exercising after a meal.[94]

People also report less fatigue and better performance if they exercise at the same time each day, according to a study published in the journal *Medical Science Sports Exercise.*[95] While this can work at any time of day, most people will find if they exercise first thing in the morning, it's easier to stick to and achieve their goals by establishing a consistent schedule.

For me, waking up and exercising immediately not only makes me feel the best, but it's also the most efficient way to use my time. I can ensure that I will make time for exercise without having to interrupt other activities to do so. And exercising first thing in the morning means you can't skip it later in the day when you get busy. Almost any kind of morning exercise, including walking, swimming, calisthenics, aerobics, or resistance training, can be part of a morning workout program.

Like our earlier ancestors, do some exercise every day within a half hour of waking and before you do anything else. This primes your body to face the day. Getting into this habit also makes it harder for other priorities to get in the way of exercise. You can choose any kind of exercise for this, from a 15-minute walk to a 45-minute swim, ten minutes of pushups and calisthenics or an hour of yoga practice. You can choose the same exercise each day or vary them. The important thing is to do *something* as soon as you wake up to prime your body for the day ahead.

Walk It Out

Here's one remarkably simple way that almost anyone can increase the amount of movement they give their body each day: go for a walk. Walking is surprisingly powerful because it is so simple. It's free. Almost anyone can do it any time, just about anywhere. It requires no equipment or preparation. You could set this book down right now and take a walk. Go ahead, the book will still be where you put it. Ten or twenty minutes from now, you will probably feel a lot better than you do now.

A recent study found that regular walking can even turn off the negative effects of certain genes.[96] Scientists know that a number of independent genes in our bodies contribute to a higher body mass index (BMI).[97] Each of us inherits some percentage of these genes. People with more of these genes activated tend to have a higher BMI than people who inherit fewer. This is one of the ways "our genes make us fat." But walking seems to down-regulate, or turn off, these genes in a significant way.

Time magazine reported on a study presented at a meeting of the American Heart Association's 2012 meeting on Epidemiology and Prevention/Nutrition, Physical Activity and Metabolism offered evidence that walking briskly for one hour per day switched off 50% of the effect of these genetic markers for higher BMI.[98] So walking doesn't just burn calories, it actually switches off, or at least turns down, the genetic signals that contribute to making you gain weight. This same study also found that sedentary daily TV watching turns the effect of these genes back on. What's really interesting is that the walking and sedentary TV watching effects were independent of each other. You could cause improvements by walking for an hour per day, but if you then spent two hours sitting around watching TV, it would negate part of that benefit. This is further evidence that it isn't enough to just get exercise. We also need to be careful of spending too much time each day in a sedentary state.

I think it's likely that, in addition to turning off the effects of some negative genes, regular walking can also turn on some genes that are beneficial to health. The hard science in this area is still very young, but we don't have to wait for definitive proof to arrive to take advantage of the obvious benefits of walking.

Because walking is so simple, it is easy to incorporate into our regular routines. Even a short walk can have great benefits, especially once you get into the habit of walking more. A study published in the *Journal of Hypertension* found that in terms of treating hypertension, both longer walks (40 minutes) and a series of shorter walks (four ten-minute walks) were effective, but that the benefits of four short walks actually lasted longer than the single long walk. Blood pressure dropped for 11 hours in total after the walks versus seven hours for those who took one continuous walk.[99]

Walking Can Beat Running

For years, walking has been seen as running's poor cousin, in terms of exercise value. While running can get you in fantastic shape and is a great exercise for many, walking is a superior exercise for many people for several reasons. First, you are more likely to suffer from a variety of injuries from running, including bad knees, twisted ankles, shin splints, and even foot problems. But because of it's much lower impact there are far fewer *walking* injuries. A lot of data available shows that for many people, habitual running can be very hard on the joints. This is especially true for people who are over their ideal weight, since the impact from running is magnified with weight.

The other reason I've long been circumspect about the benefits of habitual long-distance running is through observations in my nutrition practice. People I see who run occasionally and at moderate distances tend to be very healthy, especially if they also get other forms of exercise. I occasionally advise elite endurance athletes on nutrition, and the focus is often on using rest and nutrition to recover between runs and keeping the immune system functioning well so that no training days are lost. Habitual long-distance runners can suffer the consequences of constant pounding. I suspect that every person has an amount of running that they can recover from, both muscularly, metabolically, and in the joints and immune system. This amount varies from person to person, but if a person regularly goes over this recoverable level, they can put a strain on their bodies that mitigates some of the benefits of the physical activity to the point where regular running can actually wear a person down.

The research seems to support this view. There's mounting evidence that very high levels of endurance exercise, such as repeatedly training for and running marathons, can cause small but very real coronary damage that builds up over time.[100] [101] A study in 2011 found that lifelong marathoners had a significant level of myocardial fibrosis, the very serious and irreversible scarring of the heart valves. In fact, a shocking 50 percent of the veteran marathon runners in the study showed myocardial fibrosis, even though they showed no outward symptoms. Yet *none* of the control group of non-marathon runners of the same age were found to have myocardial fibrosis.[102]

A variety of studies show that running more than 20 miles per week may undo some of the benefits of regular exercise. A very interesting 15-year study looked at the overall mortality rates of 52,000 participants who started out with no CHD, based on their running habits. While runners did have a 19% lower risk of all-cause mortality compared to non-runners, the details were surprising. The researchers expected to find that the benefits of running would rise to a certain point and then level out, with more running not necessarily giving more benefits. However, what they actually found was the surprise. After a certain point, the mortality benefits not only leveled out, they *reversed*, meaning that more running was actually *undoing* many of the health benefits of the exercise. According to the study, the distance that conferred the lowest mortality rates was about 10-15 miles per week. That's 1.4 - 2.1 miles per day, if you walk every day. Beyond that, the benefits started to disappear. Running more than 5 days per week removed the statistical benefits entirely, as did running too fast. Runners who averaged a 6- or 7-mile per hour pace had a 27% and 21% decrease in their respective all-cause mortality, but those who ran 8-miles per hour (a 7:30 mile pace) or faster did not receive any statistical mortality benefit from running at all.[103] So running too fast, too long, or too often is clearly too much for most of us.

Source: Lee DC, Pate RR, Lavie CJ, et al. "Running and all-cause mortality risk—is more better?" *American College of Sports Medicine* 2012 Annual Meeting; June 2, 2012; San Francisco, CA. Presentation 3471.

Now, I certainly believe that some amount of running can be part of a healthy lifestyle. Research supports 10-15 total miles per week at a 8:30- to 10-minute mile pace, with at least two rest days per week.[104] This is far more than most people run today.

For most of us, walking can be a better exercise because it can be sustained longer without the negative impacts of overtraining and joint damage. A recent study supports this view. The study, published in *Arteriosclerosis, Thrombosis, and Vascular Biology* in April 2013, compared the exercise intensity and health outcomes of 33,000 runners and 16,000 walkers. Previous studies had found benefits for runners over walkers because they had compared the amount of *time* that each spent doing their activity. Because you can run farther in the same about of time than you can walk, these earlier studies found that runners get more benefit per hour spent exercising. But the new study looked at things a different way. It asked the question, "If they are traveling the same *distance*, which group of exercisers gets more benefits, walkers or runners?" For the same distance, walking and running tied on some health markers. And on the rest of the health markers, **walking proved to be almost twice as beneficial as running over the same distance.** [105]

Here are some specifics: First, the kind of walking used in the study, and the kind that I recommend for getting the maximum health benefits, is brisk walking. That means a pace of around three to five miles per hour ideally (a 12- to 20-minute per mile pace). Judging by your breathing, you should walk at a pace that's intense enough so that you can carry on a conversation, but you should not be able to sing. If you can sing a song, stop singing and pick up your pace.

Among study participants running and walking similar distances, both runners and walkers reduced the risk of diabetes by about 12% (running 12.1%, walking 12.3%); reduced hypertension by 4.2% for running and 7.2% for walking; lowered cholesterol by 4.3% for running and 7.0% for walking; and reduced CHD by 4.5% for running and 9.3% for walking. It seems that the health benefits of walking are not only "as good" as those of running, in many cases, they're better, provided you're going the same distance.

Walk This Way

Of course, to get the same distance walking as running takes nearly twice as long. Since walking in several short sessions has the same or greater benefits as one long walk each day, one great strategy is to break your daily walks up into several sessions.

Walking in the morning before breakfast is my favorite way to start the day, rain or shine, light or dark. I like to think of a morning walk as something that takes no net time, because even if I'm investing 20 or 30 minutes walking, my productivity boost over the next two to three hours makes up for the time spent walking. A morning walk is also a really easy way to knock out your exercise before breakfast.

The time after lunch and dinner is also a prime opportunity to add some walking to your schedule. Walking after a meal helps reduce the spike in triglycerides that typically follows a high-fat meal, according to a study performed in Kyoto, Japan.[106] The study found that a walk or light resistance exercise just before a meal also reduced triglyceride levels, although with a less powerful effect.

While all walking seems to show benefits, I believe that walking outside, especially in green spaces like parks and trails, has additional benefits. Trees clear the air, and the air even just a few meters inside a park can be cleaner than the air in the busy streets around its borders. The sight of trees and nature can also clear your mind. Scientists have long suspected this, but it was difficult to show because it's extremely difficult to take a stroll through the park with a huge brain scanner on your head.

A recent study performed in Scotland attached a new, lightweight form of scanner to participants. The study participants walked through green parks, pedestrian-friendly historic districts, and busy commercial areas. They found that walking in the green park area reduced the signs of mental fatigue compared to the busy area.[107] This finding is hardly surprising. Walking among trees and nature tends to calm people, increases their sense of well-being, and make them better able to focus on tasks.

How do you walk? You don't need any guidance there, right? You've been walking since you were a baby. Well, maybe some things could be changed to improve your walking. Here are a couple of suggestions. Walk with other people and consider spending some of your time walking barefoot.

Whenever possible, have a friend or loved one join you on your walk. Walking is also one of the few physical activities you can do while socializing. If you want to get closer to someone, take walks together. Not only are you both getting physical exercise and an attitude boost from being outside, but you are freed from the normal distractions that inhibit conversation. And if you typically find yourself at a loss for things to talk about, your walk can even provide that, since your constantly changing environment will offer new and unexpected topics for discussion at every turn.

Walking while socializing can make walks seem very short—sometimes too short. It often seems like you finish the walk just when the conversation gets interesting. By walking with another person, not only do you get the physical, mental, and social benefits of walking, but another person does, too.

Going Barefoot

Now for my second suggestion: walk barefoot or use the no-support "barefoot" shoes now being sold by all the major footwear companies. I realize that the very concept will strike many people as odd. Aren't we supposed to wear shoes to protect us? What about all the ads from the shoe companies? Do you believe that shoes are better for us?

Our ancestors did not evolve wearing shoes. In fact, the ancient Greeks rarely wore them. In many parts of the world today, people do not wear shoes at all. We have come to associate being barefooted with poverty or counter-culture. In America, from sneakers to wing-tips to stilettos, the shoes we wear seem to completely define our identity and social standing. But there's some surprising new thinking about the value of going barefoot over constantly wearing shoes.

When I was young, I remember my dad coming home from work every day and complaining of sore feet. My brothers and I had the job of rubbing his feet after a long day in business shoes. My lasting impression from this is of how my dad's toes had been molded together into a shape that could fit into his dress shoes. His toes were indelibly shaped by the other toes, and they fit together like nesting puzzle pieces. Even at that age, I felt this must be unnatural.

When I first traveled to Fiji, where many people do not wear shoes at all, I was struck by the difference in the shape of people's feet. Their toes spread apart, their feet were broad, and they seemed to show no discomfort at walking over jagged stone. In fact, people who do not wear shoes have very few injuries on their feet. Rarely do they even get abrasions, and bunions and fallen arches are unheard of, as these are diseases caused by wearing shoes.

Unfortunately, there's little chance that American society will change any time soon to the point where it will be acceptable to walk around barefoot as a hobbit at work or in public. However, introducing some barefoot time to your day can strengthen your feet, improve conditions like plantar fasciitis and, in my experience, reduce pain in the neck, back, and knee. The reduced joint pain is largely a product of naturally altering the way you walk while barefoot into a manner that has less impact on your joints, since you feel each step.

Of course, for feet that have spent most of their lifetime wrapped in protective shoes, barefoot walking can be quite an adjustment. The barefoot- or minimalist-style athletic shoes that reduce the amount of rubber between your foot and the ground brings some of the benefits of real barefoot walking, such as reduced joint pain and stronger feet.[108]

Another way to introduce barefoot walking is to walk in the park and take off your shoes when you reach a grassy area. Carry your shoes, and you'll feel like a kid again. Start with a hundred yards and add a little each time while your feet readjust to their natural state. And if you're lucky enough to be able to walk on a beach, kick off those flip-flops and dig your toes into the sand. Talk about a treat!

Here's another benefit to walking barefoot where the hard science is young, but is supported by anecdotal evidence and my own experience. The earth has an extremely low electrical current. This DC current varies somewhat, but it is generally negatively charged. It grounds the electrical charge of all things and beings connected to it. All living things evolved with this constant electrical grounding, including humans, of course. But wearing shoes with non-conductive soles has cut us off from this natural grounding current. When we spend time outside barefoot, we are reconnected with this grounding effect that was part of the growth of every living thing.

Being disconnected from the earth's natural grounding current and associated stream of free electrons is one cause of the free radicals in our bodies. Free radicals are unstable molecules that cause accelerated cell aging. This is similar to how they cause a cut apple to turn brown. They have a positive electrical charge that is neutralized by the low but constant negative electrical charge of the earth. This counteracts the free radicals' negative impacts on our health. Contact with the earth's electrical grounding may also help maintain an optimum pH level within our bodies. And by reducing the free radicals, it appears that oxidative stress is reduced and healing is improved. Researchers looking into the area have studied thermography, or heat images, showing that barefoot earth-grounding increases circulation throughout the body. One pilot study looked at grounding the body during sleep by using an "earthing" sheet on the bed. This was connected to the earth's current through the ground plug in the home's electrical outlet. Results included numerous reduced markers for delayed onset muscle soreness from resistance exercise, which suggests that they recovered faster and with less soreness.[109]

I sleep grounded and use the same earthing sheet from the study, and I have experienced similar benefits. I also go barefoot whenever possible, and I wear barefoot-style shoes when I walk each day and sometimes even at the office. This is a fascinating area where my personal experience validates the early scientific findings, and the research is ongoing.

So, go for walks several times a day. Walk with a friend, when possible. And slip off your shoes for part of the walk so your feet can move, too.

Sitting Is Killing You

I've always had a high need for exercise and have made it a point to get some every week. Even when work kept me the busiest, I would try to meet the minimum amount that many experts recommended, 45 minutes to an hour of exercise three times per week. Lately, however, some cutting-edge research turns the idea, and even the definition, of regular exercise on its head.

The fitness model that I, and most of America, used for the past few decades was to exercise for a total of 3-10 hours per week and then for the remainder of the 168 hours (or 112 waking hours) in a week, we go about our business certain that we had already achieved the movement needed to keep us healthy. It's a great theory, and it probably inspired a lot of people to get regular exercise. However, new research is showing that this idea isn't necessarily giving us the whole picture. How much we move or don't move during those other waking hours is important and contributes to our overall health. It may even be *more* important than our active exercise time.

Doctors have long used the word "sedentary" to describe individuals who don't get any regular exercise. By that definition, someone who *does* get regular exercise is not sedentary. However, the dictionary definition of sedentary is: *characterized by spending much time seated; not moving.*[110] In this light, even a person who spends ten hours per week exercising can be sedentary, if much of the rest of their 112 waking hours in the week are spent sitting. What researchers are finding is, even if you get the recommended amount of exercise, you still need to pay attention to the amount of time you spend in a sedentary state.[111]

Our bodies find prolonged sitting unnatural. After all, there are no chairs in nature. We evolved to move, and moving is a sign to the body that we are healthy. When we move, we burn energy. Our muscles become an important part of our circulatory system, helping to push blood throughout our bodies and deep into our tissues. From an evolutionary standpoint, sitting still for long periods of time was uncommon and probably only occurred during extended periods of food scarcity.

To our bodies, prolonged sitting may signal that it is important to conserve resources. This takes the form of several adaptations. Prolonged sitting has been found to reduce the release of lipoprotein lipase, an important enzyme that allows the body to consume fat as fuel.[112] This suggests that when we're sitting for longer than an hour, our bodies become less able to burn fat, even if we are on a reduced-calorie diet. When we're inactive, our bodies switch over to burning glucose, or blood sugar, which contributes to rising and falling blood sugar levels, which may be a precursor to diabetes. Inactivity even reduces our HDL cholesterol levels. That's the good stuff you want more of that helps clear the bad cholesterol from your system.

These responses may have helped our ancestors marshal their body's resources during lean times, but in the present day, they lead to increased risk for diabetes, heart disease, and obesity.

So is your life sedentary, even if you get several hours of exercise each week? If you sit in a car, bus, or airplane as part of your regular commute, then sit at a desk to work at a computer, and even sit in front of the TV or computer after work to unwind, then yes, you probably have a sedentary lifestyle, even if you get plenty of exercise. Is this a problem? It looks that way.

Starting in 1982, researchers at the University of South Carolina (USC) received data about a set of 7,744 healthy adult males who had been surveyed by the Cooper Clinic in Dallas, Texas, about how much sitting they did each week either driving or watching TV and also about their exercise habits. The USC researchers followed up on deaths in this group via the National Death Index through 2003 (21 years) and found that the men who sat the most (23 hours per week or more) for these activities had a 64 percent greater risk of dying from heart disease than those who sat the least (less than 11 hours per week), **regardless of the men's exercise habits**.[113] The study did find health and mortality advantages to regular exercise and being of normal weight as well. The lesson seems to be that regular exercise and time spent sitting are independent factors, and sitting too much is a strong factor in risk of death (at least in terms of cardiovascular disease), even among those who exercise regularly.

In another study published in the diabetes-related medical journal *Diabetologica*, teams in the UK looked at 18 previous studies that included a total of over 800,000 subjects. This study, led by Dr. Emma Wilmot of the University of Leicester, found that **those people who sat the most had *double* the risk for diabetes, plus a higher risk for heart disease and death compared to those test subjects who sat the least**.[114] And according to another study, published in the *International Journal of Behavioral Nutrition and Physical Activity*, this is true even of people who regularly exercise.[115]

I think there is often reason to be cautious about results from new studies. Sometimes they use small sample sizes or look at an issue in a way that future studies may modify or invalidate. However, rather than performing original tests, a "survey study" such as this takes a fresh look at existing data and compares it across several different studies. A survey study looks at similar issues across different populations to see what can be learned. When I see results from a survey study, I tend to find it quite persuasive, especially if a large number of studies and subjects are involved. And 800,000 subjects from 18 peer-reviewed studies is a very large sample size. So this is a study with some real power behind it.

What does this mean? On the face of it, it means that the people from each study who spent the most time sitting had twice the risk of getting diabetes compared to the people from each study who spent the least time sitting each day. This group's risk for heart disease and death was also higher. That all sounds kind of scary. But I think there's a better way to look at it. The way I see it, **if you are in a lifestyle that has you sitting for several hours each day, then you may currently be at a higher risk for diabetes and heart disease. But you can significantly cut those risks, starting right now, by simply standing up and stepping out of that group.**

How do you remove yourself from this group that has such startling health implications? Stand up! You might want to do it right now. You have the power in this scenario. If you don't want to be sedentary, the solution is to stand up. Hey, look at you: You're not sedentary anymore.

It can't really be that simple, can it? *Maybe it can!* Another study published in the journal *BMJ Open*, found that limiting the amount of time Americans spent sitting each day to a total of just three hours could increase that average life expectancy by up to two years.[116]

Don't Take This Sitting Down!

Here's a very simple solution to the problem of excessive sitting. Stand up! As the repercussions of too much sitting have become known, stand-up desks have grown popular. I started using a stand-up desk four years ago. I immediately felt an improvement in my circulation and well-being, compared to sitting all day. However, it's a big change, and you don't have to switch over from sitting to standing all day to start feeling the benefits. I find that a blend is best.

When I started using my stand-up desk, I split my time 50-50 between sitting and standing. That helped me get used to standing more throughout my day. It also meant that I wasn't sitting for hours at a time. This let me adjust gradually to standing. After several months, I was up to standing for about 75% of my workday, which is my current practice. Standing for most of my day has made huge differences in the way my back, neck, and shoulders feel at the end of the work day. Who knew that sitting could make me feel so tired? At the end of a long day of sitting, I used to go home and sit some more, just to recover.

Of course, standing for much of the day can take some getting used to, so start gradually. Alternating is a great strategy, and be sure to work more movement into your workday so you are not standing in one place all day.

Movement Is the Key

The best way to combat a sedentary lifestyle is by adding more movement. Researchers call general movement, which is less than exercise but more than sitting, non-exercise physical activity (NEPA). Typically, NEPA is walking, doing housework, gardening, moving furniture, and the like. And it turns out that NEPA has a big impact on our health and fitness. In a study published in 2014 in the *British Journal of Sports Medicine*, researchers followed 4,232 60-year old subjects for an average of 12.5 years and found that the high-NEPA group had more preferable waist circumferences, HDL levels, and triglyceride levels in both men and women and lower insulin and glucose levels in men compared to the low-NEPA group. This was all regardless of what other exercise the subjects performed.[117]

At home, getting more movement, or NEPA, can mean playing with your kids, walking a pet, doing some yard work or household chores, almost anything where you're not sitting or standing in one place for long periods. In the office, that can mean walking to meetings or spending some time at a stand-up desk. You can purchase a stand-up desk that's ready-made, or you can improvise by stacking boxes on your desktop. Some people are using treadmill desks or even adding laptop trays to treadmills to create walking desks. However, simpler strategies can also yield good results. You can march in place at a stand-up desk, or even fidget to increase the amount of movement you do in a day.

Other approaches for getting you up off your behind:

- Have stand-up meetings where no one sits down. Not only does this increase everyone's movement level, but it often leads to shorter, more productive meetings.
- Walk to co-workers' desks instead of sending email. This gets you some exercise and can often help you quickly discuss and resolve a matter that might have taken several exchanged messages back and forth.
- Stand up for phone calls. I've been doing this for years and have noticed a very clear connection between standing and a positive outcome of the call. Not only can you get more movement this way, but people's voices tend to sound more authoritative when they're standing up.
- Inflatable therapy balls can be a great alternative to an office chair. In one study, researchers found that a therapy ball also increased the number of calories people burned in an hour compared to sitting in a normal office chair. [118]

Exercise the "Off" Button

For years, doctors and medical researchers have assumed that watching too much TV had an adverse affect on people's health. But no one ever tried to put a number to how much impact it was having. Well, a group of researchers in Queensland, Australia, compared data from the Australian Bureau of Statistics with the Australian Diabetes, Obesity, and Lifestyle study to see if they could figure out, statistically, just what effect an hour of watching TV had on a person's health. Their results, published in the *British Journal of Sports Medicine*, were staggering: **For an adult over 25, one hour of watching TV statistically shortens the viewer's life by 22 minutes.**[119]

More than one-third of the time you spend sitting and watching TV is time that you are literally shaving off your life expectancy. I hope it's a great show!

How big is this problem? According to the 2012 Neilson surveys, the average American over age 2 watches 34 hours of TV per week.[120] Based on the study's findings, this would mean that the average American is shortening his or her life by 27 days each year due to sedentary TV-watching. **That's about one entire month that's being slashed from your life every single year. For TV!** Maybe even re-runs! We are literally sitting our lives away.

Even setting aside the grave health issues associated with sitting to watch TV, the life-wasting side of it also is important. Americans watch an average of 34 hours of TV per week. That's an insane amount, nearly a day and a half each week, and it doesn't even include the amount of Internet surfing, YouTube viewing, and Facebook browsing that Americans have added to their lives in the past few years.

Sedentary, passive consumption of media in mass amounts has become one of the biggest chunks of time in our waking lives. Many people spend more time glued to a screen than they do working. If this sounds like you, consider how much happier you will be and how much more time you will have to spend with your loved ones, how much you can improve your health, how much you can advance your career or how much you can help with causes, simply by exercising one finger and pushing the Off button on your TV or computer. Please don't waste your leisure time watching hours of TV or mindless Internet videos.

If you are typical, cutting your TV and recreational Internet time down to one hour per day would give you back more than 27 hours every week. That's enough to add 90 minutes of exercise, an extra hour of sleep, and plenty of additional *real* social time with family, friends, or co-workers every day of the week. And you'd probably have extra time left over to read a book before bed. Think how much richer your life could be just by watching less TV.

If you are wondering how you can possibly accommodate the additional exercise, sleep, and other activities that this book recommends into your already busy life, I have a simple suggestion that will suddenly make everything fit. Stop watching TV and browsing Facebook and YouTube for more than one hour per day. Suddenly, you will have more than enough time to focus on these activities and other aspects of life that you've been missing. So exercise the Off button. Limit TV and recreational Internet use to one hour per day. That ought to be plenty to indulge in the shows you *actually* like rather than just whatever's on. You'll probably find that you can sleep better, concentrate more completely, and enjoy your life more fully. Your life is about to get a whole lot better.

The Fountain of Youth Is a Pool

In 1513 Juan Ponce de León traveled to Florida to search for the Fountain of Youth, a mystical body of water that would stave off aging and maintain good health in those who bathed in its waters. While he may not have found what he was after, I believe I have. In fact, the fountain of youth is in my own back yard. And it may be in your yard or community too. It turns out the fountain of youth may be a swimming pool.

If you asked me to recommend one exercise that would be best for just about everyone at almost any stage of life, my answer would be a very clear and simple choice: swimming. Walking may be the easiest activity to do at any time, but swimming appears to be the all-around healthiest.

Of course, it's best to get a variety of types of exercise and activity. But after looking at the research and empirical evidence, I've come to believe that swimming has benefits that no other exercise can match. That's why for my own health, the exercise I do more than any other is swimming.

Swim Yourself 20 Years Younger

People who swim regularly have the health markers of someone 20 years younger than their actual age. This is based on health data collected from hundreds of Masters swimmers and compared to the general population. The paper, presented to the World Sports Medicine Congress by Dr. Joel Stager, found that in terms of blood pressure, cholesterol levels, cardiovascular fitness, and central nervous system and cognitive functioning, the habitual swimmers in the study had health functions of people much younger.[121] [122]

These swimmers, ranging from age 20 to 86, swam 3,500 to 5,000 yards three to five times per week. This is 70-100 lengths per session in an Olympic-sized pool. In doing so, they were significantly postponing the biological aging process and building or maintaining more muscle mass than the general population. Other studies have shown that swimming 45 minutes a day, three times per week, significantly lowered blood pressure in people with hypertension, compared to a similar control group.[123] [124] I expect that, like other exercise, swimming also helps to lower weight and the risk of diabetes and cardiovascular disease as well.

Okay, so swimming regularly has a lot of benefits. What makes it better than other forms of exercise? To me, the answer lies in the specific benefits of swimming that no other exercise can claim.

First is easy access. Most communities in the U.S. have at least a public pool or YMCA, so find out where it is and join! Once you have a place to swim, you don't need much beyond a swimsuit and goggles.

Swimming is a total body exercise. Swimming laps engages the core, arms, legs, chest, lats, and back—all the major muscles in the body. Consider swimmers like Michael Phelps. They have very proportionate bodies compared to athletes like skaters or cyclists, where certain muscles dominate.

Swimming is a no-impact activity, so it spares the joints compared to activities like running, where constant pounding can lead to problems. At the same time, the water provides constant, moderate resistance from every angle. Swimming forces you to concentrate on your breathing, as in yoga or meditation. Cognitive benefits may also fit this focus. The water's constant temperature prevents overheating in hot climates. For many people, going for a run in the desert Southwest and similar climates in summer is just asking for heat stroke. And perhaps most important, swimming is fun. It often feels more like play than exercise.

I think a couple of these points are worth a closer look. Because water is about 800 times more dense than air, when we move through it, we encounter moderate resistance at every angle, not just downwards like with weightlifting. So swimming is not only a cardiovascular workout, it's a light resistance workout as well. This resistance, however, comes with zero impact, so it doesn't punish joints the way that running does. These facts combine to make swimming a fantastic form of recovery from other injuries, overtraining, or long periods of inactivity. Although the resistance is light, it builds up over the course of a workout. As a swimmer grows to move faster, the resistance increases, along with swimming ability, because trying to move faster in water creates greater resistance.

As a result, swimming and other water-based exercises have been found to improve the use of arthritis-affected joints without worsening symptoms.[125] [126] In fact, people with rheumatoid arthritis have been found to gain more health benefits from swimming than other activities, according to a study published in the journal *Arthritis Care and Research*.[127] Another study finds that in older people, swimming has been found to improve quality of life and reduce disability. It also maintains or even improves bone density for post-menopausal women.[128] [129] These are profound benefits.

All this science is very persuasive, but I can't help but feel that one of the greatest benefits of swimming is how much fun it can be. I grew up swimming in a small lake in Washington state. The weather was cold most of the year, so we had only about four months when we could swim in Lake Sammamish. But my brothers and I pushed the season every spring to get in the water. And we spent most of our summers with our heads bobbing in the lake's clear waters. Now, decades and tens of thousands of pool laps later, I still can't completely separate my swimming time from those memories of childhood fun when "exercise" was really "having a great time." This is my hope for myself, my friends, and you, that exercise can stop being a chore or an appointment or anything we do primarily to get healthy and instead reverts to that blissful state of play, enjoyment, competition, and bliss that we all had as children.

Ever see a kid in a bouncy house at a birthday party? That kid is probably burning 800 calories an hour and having the time of his life. That's joyful exercising and joyful living. And for me, the nostalgia, buoyancy, and flat-out fun of swimming gets me closer to that state than anything I could possibly put into my calendar five or so days per week.

I'm not alone in seeing the benefits of swimming to a person's sense of well-being. Swimming, like yoga, has been shown to reduce feelings of anger, confusion, depression, and tension in both men and women, according to a study published in the journal *Perceptual Motor Skills*.[130] For women, yoga and swimming showed roughly equal benefits. I expect more research will be performed in this area, but it certainly meshes with my experience.

If you're convinced that swimming can offer some very real advantages to your heath and well-being, what's the best way to incorporate it into your life?

Swim! Get in a pool and start swimming. If you are just starting, use a mask and snorkel for the first few weeks to get a feel for it. I recommend booking a set amount of time in the pool, say, 30 minutes. Swim for the first few minutes, then just move in the water for the rest of the time. It's fun, and once you have the habit, you will gradually build up the strength and endurance to swim for the entire 30 minute "appointment."

If you're new to swimming, or returning after a long break, start out with one 30-minute session every week. If that's too much time to swim, simply stay in the pool moving for the full 30 minutes to form the habit. Add more swimming as your body adjusts. After two to three months of regular swimming, you could work up to three to four times per week at 30-45 minutes per session. This is the level of swimming that has shown benefits in many of the studies.

If you're someone who is already quite active with exercise, you could replace a few of your regular workouts with swimming. Not only will you maintain your cardiovascular exercise, but you'll add resistance—all while giving your joints a few more days off each week to recover. Adding swimming to your fitness regimen will also give you a new challenge, which can help shake up stale workouts and offer even accomplished exercisers new dimensions of fitness.

Whether you're new to swimming, returning after a break, or adding it to an already regular workout program, be careful about overdoing it. Swimming faster than a moderate pace may not confer any additional benefits, since it tends to shorten workouts. Slow and steady wins the swimming race, at least while you're still adjusting to this program.

What about people who don't like swimming laps or who don't yet have the confidence in their swimming ability? Well, there's good news here. Water aerobics are a popular option for many people who want to exercise in the pool without necessarily swimming laps. There's evidence that water aerobics may give benefits similar to lap swimming.[131,132] The zero-impact resistance/cardio training is still there. So if you prefer this, then go for it. Do what you enjoy.

Here's more good news about swimming: due to water's higher density, a 30-minute workout in the pool may be equivalent to 45 minutes of similar exercise on dry land. So the pool is actually even more time efficient.

Seek Salt Water

Whenever possible, find a pool that uses a salt water or saline system, instead of chlorine. For years, pools used chemicals like chlorine and pH balancers to kill bacteria and remain sanitary. While these chemicals helped prevent the transmission of disease, they could be quite harsh. They killed germs by creating a percentage of toxic chlorine gas molecules, which don't do us humans a whole lot of good. (See Pillar Five: Hosting Well for more information about the importance of avoiding chlorine.)

Saline systems are becoming more prevalent. They still use a very small amount of chlorine to kill germs, but it is a tiny fraction of what a chlorine pool uses. Because saline pools use salts to keep bacteria in check, they need a lot less chlorine to kill the bugs. That's great for all the people swimming in the pool as well. So if you have a choice, go to a saline pool or encourage your local pool to switch over. This is a growing movement in communities across the country. If this isn't possible, the benefits of regular swimming seem to be worth the chlorine exposure. Just be sure to shower off well after a swim.

For me, the ultimate place to swim is in the ocean near my home in southeast Florida, where it is warm enough to swim year round. There's nothing like sharing your swim with reef fish and the occasional manatee!

Grounded by Water

Remember the benefits of earth-grounding I mentioned in the walking section? Well, because water is highly conductive and your entire body is immersed, swimming grounds your body much better than even barefoot walking. This grounding effect is most pronounced in ocean water, because the high ion level makes it the best conductor. Saline pools also exhibit this enhanced conductivity, though at a lower level than sea water. This grounding effect is one of the reasons that you feel great at the beach. Through swimming, wading in the sea, or walking barefoot along the strand, you are rapidly reconnecting your body to the natural current of the earth.

Swimming truly is the fountain of youth. Find a nearby pool (hopefully saline, rather than chlorine), lake, or lagoon, and jump in and start swimming. The cardiovascular and muscle benefits of swimming are profound, and because of the buoyancy and resistance of water, swimming gives you these benefits without much risk of repetitive injuries the way running can. Swim three to five times a week for 30-45 minutes, and you will see real improvements in your ability to move well.

Standing, walking, and swimming will add movement to your life, but you need more. You need muscle! Increasing the amount of muscle you have has real and significant health benefits. Of course, muscle makes you stronger in terms of being able to lift and carry more, but it also increases your strength and coordination in lots of little ways that you'll begin to notice and enjoy as your muscle mass grows. Muscle mass and strength have been found to be the single strongest indicator of five-year survival from all causes and especially from cancer, according to a nearly 20-year study of 8,762 men aged 20-80.[133] In fact, muscle mass was a far better predictor than BMI. Having more muscle also gives you more energy and helps to buffer your hormones and blood sugar levels better. And since muscle burns more energy every minute of the day, having more muscle helps keep you at a healthier weight, even when you're not actively exercising.

In fact, almost all of the things that people associate with youth, health, and well-being can be achieved or improved by increasing the amount of muscle you have. Now, a lot of people think it isn't possible to add more muscle after a certain age. But they're wrong. The science shows conclusively that with the proper exercise program, anyone at any age can build muscle mass.

It's interesting to note that some of the most brilliant minds studying these topics are also some of the most fit. My friend Dr. Jeff Stout is a famous researcher on skeletal muscle. He happens to be built like the football players he studies. Another friend, Dr. Jose Antonio, is a world-famous exercise physiologist who works with some of the top endurance athletes in the world. He recently took up outrigger canoeing and gained at least a couple of inches around his shoulders. These guys know the benefits of exercise, and they practice what they preach.

So how do we add muscle mass? Swimming is a light resistance exercise and will build some muscle. But to really get the kind of results that will make a positive impact on your health, you need to incorporate resistance training into your schedule.

What Is Resistance Training?

Resistance training, very simply, is pushing or pulling against a force that resists your efforts and makes you exert yourself. That force could be a weight machine at the gym, elastic bands, hand weights, or even your own body weight. Virtually all the things we associate with youth, health, and well-being can be achieved or improved through resistance training: more strength and coordination; better bone density and hormonal levels; lower incidence of falls. Muscle mass even helps protect people in falls or accidents by cushioning bones and organs from some of the impact. Resistance training improves mental focus and relieves stress, improves the immune system, combats diabetes and high blood sugar, raises levels of testosterone and insulin-like growth factor-I (IGF-I, a growth factor associated with health), and reduces arthritis and improves joint health. The benefits are profound.

At this point, a lot of people may be thinking, "Sure, that's great if you've stayed in shape your whole life. But what if you haven't?" If you're out of shape, overweight, or maybe have stiff joints and less mobility than you'd like, is it really worth it to start resistance training?

Yes.

Actually, what I mean is: *YES!*

Time and again, science has shown that it is not too late. Maybe it's *never* too late to increase your strength. And if you're not already exercising, you are likely to start seeing results even earlier than you may expect.

In a program called the Tufts Strong Living Program, several volunteers over age 60 were able to *double* their leg strength with a moderate resistance training and conditioning program. But more impressive: some people in the program over the age of 90 were able to stop using a cane to walk due to their increased strength, conditioning, and coordination from this program. That is a real and marked improvement in their lives. And you can bet that their increased mobility and quality of life didn't stop at walking. Increased muscle makes everything easier, so getting up out of a chair or bed, carrying things, even standing was likely much easier and more enjoyable for the volunteers in this study.[134]

When we engage in resistance training, our muscles respond by increasing protein synthesis (that's science lingo for "building muscle"), modifying our hormone production to be more like that of a younger person, and even stimulating new satellite cells—the "stem cells" of muscle tissue. These changes happen even on a low-protein diet, but eating plenty of good protein can improve your results.

How long does it take to see results? Well, two recent studies found that resistance training can begin building measurable new muscle mass in as little as two weeks. And these studies weren't just of younger people. They included subjects ages 78-84, 23-32, and 76-79.[135] [136]

Have you ever wondered why, as you get older, you have to eat less just to maintain your current weight? Well, the answer has a scientific name: sarcopenia. Every year after about the age of 30, the average American loses one half pound of muscle mass. This leads to a loss of around three to five percent of our muscle mass every decade. This insidious process is known as sarcopenia, and over time the loss of muscle mass leads to a slowdown of our metabolic rate. That means that you burn fewer calories than you used to when doing the same things, and that contributes to weight gain. Muscle loss, metabolic slowdown, and weight gain can become a vicious circle. Most Americans are well aware of this fact, either from their own lives or those of others around them.

The good news is that sarcopenia and its results can be slowed and even partially reversed through resistance training.

Resistance training is, simply put, pushing or pulling against a resisting force. That force could be a weight machine at the gym, elastic bands, hand weights, or even your own body weight. Many programs are available, but the good news is that almost any of these will help you build muscle and resist sarcopenia.

Exactly *what* resistance training program you do is a lot less important than that you *do* it, and do it regularly. Enjoyment and accessibility are key here, because if you find a program that you like and can do easily, then you are much more likely to keep doing it. And that's where you'll get the results. Some people like body weight exercises like pushups and lunges, others enjoy free weights, and for some, gym machines or elastic bands feel more accessible. Great! Do what you like.

How much resistance training should you get? One very easy way to approach it is "3-4-5." That's three sessions per week of about 45 minutes each. This 45 minutes should include a warm up of around ten minutes and a cool down of about ten minutes of light stretching. And between them, include about 30 minutes of resistance training. If you're doing resistance training three times per week, then you will probably see the best results if you hit all the major muscle groups every session. That's legs, back, chest, arms, and core. Some people prefer to do resistance training four times per week and split up muscle groups, training upper-body and lower body, or else the "push" muscles (chest, triceps, etc.) and "pull" muscles (back, biceps, etc.) on alternating workouts. That's fine, too. Remember, these are minimums. You can always do more once you get into a groove, but if you're new to resistance training, 3-4-5 is probably a pretty good place to start.

Where do these numbers come from? Well, they're similar to the protocols used in many of the studies. Not coincidentally, some variation on this mix are also found in many popular workout programs. Three times per week for 30 minutes or more seems to be the amount of resistance exercise that provides effective muscle building without being too demanding on our bodies or schedules.

This is a manageable amount for most people. However, some people *love* resistance training, especially once they start seeing results. It's an amazing feeling to know that you are building strength, muscle, and coordination, that you can do things that you couldn't do a few weeks ago (and building up "youth hormones" in the process). For some, it's tempting to overdo it. This can lead to better results, but it can also lead to burnout. So, like anything new, ease into it. Spend three to four months in the 3-4-5 zone before you expand your program. Remember, this is something you're adding for life. There's no need to rush it.

By that same token, it's important to look around at programs and exercises until you find something that you really enjoy doing. The more you enjoy an exercise program, the more likely you are to actually do it, and the more fun you'll have while doing it. The goal is to improve your life and health by incorporating healthier *lifelong* habits. So choosing something you really enjoy goes a long way.

An absolute wealth of options is available to you. Dozens of great workout programs are available on DVD. Your local gym, fitness center, or parks department likely has numerous resistance training classes you could take. You can lift weights with a group of friends or do a routine from one of the hundreds of books available. But which one is best? Who cares!

There's really no point in trying to figure out which resistance training is best. Just as almost everyone rates themselves an "above average" driver, most exercise plans claim to be best or better than the others. The "best" program is the one that's best for you, the one you will actually do. Think about it this way: let's say one of these programs is better than all the others. Even if that was true, you'll still get about 95% of the same benefits of resistance training just by doing *any* program (within the 3-4-5 guidelines). So at most, you're missing out on maybe 5% potential benefits. Big deal. Doing the exercise is what's important, plus having fun doing it. Small hand weights are great. Elastic's fantastic. Slow lifting works great for people.

Like walking, you can do your resistance training with other people to make it even more fun. People stick with their workouts more when they make an appointment that includes others. Everyone has days when it's tough to get started exercising. Myself included, though I find that once I actually start, I tend to love doing it, and I'm left wondering why it was so hard to get rolling. Knowing that someone else is expecting you, or that you're paying for a session with a trainer that you are missing, can help you stick with it on those tougher days. So work out with a friend when you can. Start a program together, and you'll both benefit from it.

Personal trainers can also help you stick with a program. More importantly, a trainer can teach you the proper form for exercise, assess your weaknesses, and create a program that you're likely to enjoy and get better results from while avoiding injury. If you're new to resistance training, I highly recommend that you work with a trainer for your first six sessions or so to get you up and running. Think of this as 3-4-5-6. After these first two weeks, you can either continue with the trainer if that works best for you, or else go on your own, checking in every four to six months or so to assess your progress, correct any mistakes, and update your program.

Stretch Your Health Span

Until a few years ago, I never appreciated the value of a good stretch. I'd seen my cat do it ten times a day and knew that some of the serious athletes I work with swear it helps them feel and perform better. But I was sticking with weights, running, and hitting the punching bag. Then in my early–40s, my back began to hurt badly enough that I sought medical attention with an osteopathic doctor. He told me to try stretching first and gave me an at-home prescription. It took about two months of twice-daily stretching for 15 minutes at a time before I started to loosen up, but then what a difference! Yoga and Pilates sessions are even more powerful, and by the time I was 46, I was able to touch my toes without bending my legs for the first time in my adult life. Now at 50-plus I'm free from back pain as long as I keep up with stretching twice a day for about ten minutes per session. Yogis since the dawn of civilization have told us that staying flexible equals staying young, and now I believe them.

Supplement Support

When it comes to simply moving well every day, no supplements are necessary. Just get out there and move! However, if you want to safely increase your energy for a workout or speed your muscle recovery afterwards, a few clinically supported supplements are worth taking.

Niagen® NR: Mitochondrial Energy Booster

The first supplement is a specific metabolite of vitamin B_3 called nicotinamide riboside (NR), brand named Niagen®. This occurs in very small amounts in foods like milk. In addition, NR is a metabolic precursor of nicotinamide adenine dinucleotide (NAD), required by the mitochondria in all human cells for production of energy within the cell. Our bodies easily convert Niagen to NAD.

This is important, because all the energy that your cells use comes from your mitochondria. They are literally the powerhouses for our bodies. Each cell in your body can have anywhere from two mitochondria to two thousand, depending on age, type, and condition. The more mitochondria a cell has, and the better shape they're in, the more energy they can produce.

But like everything, mitochondria need the right conditions to give their best.

Every cell in our bodies relies on its mitochondria for energy, and mitochondria need NAD. So, NR is an efficient precursor for NAD production, and that fuels up our mitochondria. The NAD levels can drop as we age, possibly reducing the natural energy production. Yet NAD helps keep mitochondria functioning at their best for natural energy production, without artificial stimulation of the central nervous system. In addition, NAD can help build a better athlete from the inside, supporting energy and fitness at the cellular level.

I take 100 mg of Niagen NR daily, which is the clinically studied dose shown to boost NAD levels by up to 2.7-fold in a human trials.[137]

Creatine: Muscle Cell Energy

Creatine is a substance that exists in every cell of our bodies and is a crucial part of the muscle cell's energy cycle. In fact, our own bodies create creatine. However, it's been known since the early 20th century that supplementing with additional creatine can increase athletic performance. Creatine works by making muscle cells work more efficiently. Creatine also increases the activity of satellite cells, the stem cells of muscle tissue that are responsible for building new muscle cells.[138]

Various studies have also found creatine can increase levels of testosterone, dihydrotestosterone, and insulin-like growth factor-I (IGF-I), all positive changes to your hormonal system that mimic the state we are in when we're younger. [139] [140]

To get the benefits of creatine supplementation, I recommend taking creatine monohydrate, which is the least expensive form. It has recently been shown to be just as effective as other forms, like buffered creatine.[141] Taking two to five grams of creatine monohydrate daily, mixed with water or juice, is enough to get the benefits for most people.

I take mine before lifting weights, in plain water. It takes a bit of stirring to get it to dissolve, but it doesn't have any flavor. It does, however, have a slightly gritty texture if you don't get it all stirred in.

If you have renal disease, it may be better to skip creatine, as some studies indicate it may increase the chance of kidney dysfunction in people who already have renal problems. However, there's no evidence to show that it causes harm in otherwise healthy individuals, and mounting evidence indicates that it may do a lot of good.[142]

Branched-chained amino acids (BCAAs) are naturally occurring compounds that are already in our diets, to some extent. Scientists have found that taking BCAAs as supplements can significantly increase the benefits of exercise, particularly resistance training.

Amino acids are the building blocks of all protein. Twenty-one different kinds of amino acids exist, and they combine in various patterns to make every type of protein there is. Of these, nine are "essential" amino acids that our bodies cannot create on their own and that must come from our diet. Three of these—leucine, valine, and isoleucine–are "branched-chain amino acids" that are believed to significantly increase muscle growth over resistance training alone. [143] In addition, BCAAs have also been found to reduce muscle soreness after training.[144]

To get the benefits of BCAAs, you can either take isolated BCAA supplements or food that is rich in BCAAs. Supplements may be more trouble and expense than other options, like whey protein powder or a protein blend that includes whey protein. When Little Miss Muffet sat on her tuffet, eating her curds and whey, she was really eating what we'd call cottage cheese. The watery part is whey and has a protein in it called whey protein, which is very high in BCAAs. The curd part contains cheese protein, called casein. Both of these are found in milk. Taking a powdered protein supplement can get a lot of BCAAs into your system very quickly. But then, so can eating come cottage cheese, yogurt, or any dairy product, and probably at less expense. In fact, chocolate milk has been found to be an ideal recovery drink after resistance training (but watch the sugar content). Some research suggests that a mix of proteins, like whey and casein, which are found in natural dairy products, is better at promoting muscle growth than pure whey protein.[145]

On days when you do resistance training, aim to have some BCAAs 15 minutes before your workout and a half hour afterwards, then again in the evening. This has been found to increase the effects of resistance training, improve muscle repair after workouts and help build more muscle.

PRESCRIPTION № 3

1. Move Before You Eat

2. Stand Up For Your Health

3. Lift A Little

4. Exercise the Off Button

5. Swim for Life

6. Stay Flexible

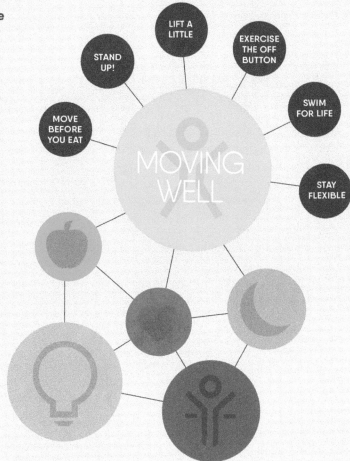

Moving is one of the great joys in life, and our bodies were designed to move every day. While our modern conveniences have eliminated much of the physical work from daily life, that's exactly what most of us need to stay healthy and fit. The good news is that we can add back exercise when and how we choose, so instead of chasing down game or lifting bales of hay all day we can take a walk or a swim and lift some weights and call it good. Establishing daily habits and routines are the most powerful tools in this arsenal, so move every single day whether you "feel like it" right then or not. In the real world, your energy levels, the weather, and the time demands of work and daily life will be variable. When tradeoffs are inevitable, don't skip a day moving your body. It is far more important to be fanatical about consistency than intensity. Do something each day. Staying consistent in all weather and conditions also reinforces the positive habit of daily movement, which pays dividends in all other facets of Living Well.

1. Move Before You Eat

Daily walking is simple and free and offers a panacea of proven health benefits. Walking for 20-30 minutes before you eat ensures you won't skip it and kicks off a positive cascade of hormones and endorphins that make your whole day more productive. The research indicates that 10-15 miles a week (so about 1.5 miles per day) is the optimal for health and longevity. The belief that getting a few hours of exercise each week will make up for sitting for hours on end the rest of the time is proving to be misguided. For optimum health, it's important to not only get exercise and but also reduce the amount of time you spend sitting.

2. Stand Up For Your Health

Don't take a desk job sitting down! Even if you are at a computer terminal all day, raise it to standing eye level, and you will feel the difference almost immediately. Long periods of inactivity throughout the day have a very harsh effect on our fitness and well-being. It's not reasonable to expect that a few hours of exercise will make up for sitting around the rest of the day. Find ways to break up long periods of sitting by standing up, walking around, and even performing a few stretches and exercises when you can. Modify your workspace if possible so that you have the option of standing for part of your day. The best solution is an adjustable desk that can be used either sitting or standing. I use the VariDesk, made by an Australian company. Remember, sitting is the new smoking in terms of health risk, so stand up for your health.

3. Lift a Little

Resistance training with weights has been proven to benefit almost every age group studied, from teenagers to the very elderly. I recommend buying your own weights or bands so that the weight room is always nearby. Unless you are training to be a competitive athlete, do a set of lifting exercises that work every major muscle group no more than three times a week, with at least one rest day between to let your muscles recover. Once you get past an initial soreness period, this is a workout to look forward to with enormous benefits in strength, health, weight management, and longevity.

Your thumb flexor can be the most important muscle you exercise each day by turning off the TV to free up time to exercise. Watching TV and, increasingly, viewing social media and video sites on the Internet not only increases your daily sitting time, but it takes away precious hours that you could spend in more meaningful and positive ways such as getting adequate sleep, exercising, or spending real in-person time with others. For some reason, TVs seem much easier to turn on than they are to turn off, even though it's all the same button. This is especially true if you are watching more out of habit or boredom than a deep interest in the program you're watching. Exercise the Off button and take back your time for more beneficial and enjoyable uses. Getting off the couch is the single most important fitness step many of us can take, and with an average 3.8 hours a day spent in front of the TV, there's plenty of time in there for a 30-minute workout.

The fountain of youth is a swimming pool, and chances are good that there's one nearby. Join it if you can and spend a half hour there three or more times a week. If you're not already a strong swimmer, I recommend going to the pool for 30 minutes to establish the habit. Splash around, take a lap or two, kick against the wall in the shallow end, or walk around in the water. Once you get in the habit of going to the pool, you will eventually build up to a daily swim and the benefits of the real Fountain of Youth.

Stretching is absolutely free, and it's one of the best daily habits you can adopt for feeling younger and more flexible with fewer aches and pains. Start slow and don't push past the point of gentle tension on the muscle.

I've found something magical about stretching right when you wake up, like my cat does, and then again right before bedtime. This helps me become more flexible and reduces lower back pain.

SLEEPING WELL

"Sleep is the best meditation."

—Dalai Lama

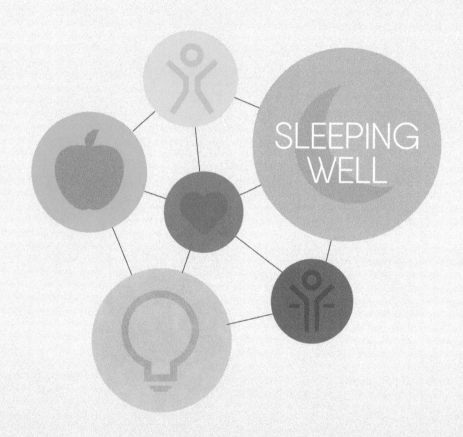

SLEEPING WELL

SLEEPING WELL

What if I told you that there was something you could do for free that required no effort and only took an hour? And what if it was scientifically proven beyond a doubt to improve your mood, make you measurably more productive in your job, help you control your appetite, could detoxify your brain and give you better cognitive skills, might reduce your chances of getting in an accident, and would even make you sexier? You'd do it in a minute, right?

Since we were children, our parents have told us to get plenty of sleep. And time and again the research is proving mom right. Getting less than eight hours of sleep very quickly impairs our productivity, judgment, health, and even our safety. Insufficient sleep undercuts everything we do in other areas of our lives: health, weight loss, career, and relationships. And yet, as a nation we have a sleep debt that rivals our national debt. A 2013 Gallup study found that two-thirds of American adults average less than seven hours of sleep per night and over half of adults under 50 say they would feel better with more sleep.[146] So, on average, every night we all get a little deeper into a sleep debt that leaves us groggy, moody, less productive, and more accident prone.

What can we do about this? The good news is that simply getting the right amount of sleep each night can quickly remedy the problem. Getting eight hours of sleep for several nights in a row can rejuvenate your mind and give you better focus. It can also have a profound effect on your body. Many people who find themselves stuck in a rut in terms of fitness, weight loss, and happiness discover that simply getting enough sleep each night helps them easily break free from their former roadblocks. This makes sense, because often what's holding us back is exhaustion.

Animals do not have sleeping problems. They simply sleep. Have you ever admired the depth of slumber achieved by a cat? Mine is a vicious killer of rodents and lizards in our neighborhood for a few hours each day. The rest of the time, he is curled up in a comfortable spot in a state of total bliss. Sleeping well means not just quantity but quality of sleep, and making some simple changes can help you sleep like an animal.

Sleep: Your Biological Need

Why do *all* mammals sleep? The question has intrigued researchers for decades. We know that depriving mammals of sleep results in reduced capacity to think, to react to stimuli, and to control appetite.[147] It also eventually leads to an earlier death. [148] So, there is no doubt that sleep is critical to good health in mammals, including humans. But why do we sleep at all? It seems like such a waste of time to shut down many of our mental and physical processes for several hours every day. If some other band of humans could have evolved to need no sleep, wouldn't they have taken over while our own sleep-needing ancestors were dozing?

Scientists have had many theories over the years about *why* we sleep. Early thoughts on the subject were based around ideas of conserving energy and staying out of harm's way. In other words, it was simply a way to not burn precious calories and keep from attracting predators. We call this hibernation. But there are some holes in this theory. Even hibernating animals need to wake up from hibernation to sleep! Arctic ground squirrels have been found to wake up for periods of hibernation so that they can get sleep.[149] Even animals like dolphins that need to be awake to keep breathing still sleep—they've just evolved to allow one hemisphere of their brain to sleep at a time so that they don't drown. And as far as we know, no animal except for man has sleeping problems or voluntarily short-changes sleep for other waking activities.

Detoxifying the Brain

Recent research has helped to clear up the mystery of why we sleep. Brain cells have a very taxing function. So much so, in fact, that it appears that they are not able to do their work *and* clear out the toxic by-products of their metabolism at the same time. This is different than most other cells in our bodies. Our heart cells, for example, need to keep operating without a break every second for our entire lives. Other muscle cells tend to clear their wastes while they operate, except when pushed into overdrive by a big predator or, perhaps a particularly challenging spin or kickboxing class. In this overdrive mode, the muscles go full-out until we choose to stop (we escape the bear), or until too many toxic metabolic by-products like lactic acid build up in the muscle and impair its function, reducing our ability to run or even cramping our muscles. Then they need to clear out these waste products after the high-intensity exercise is done. This is part of why your muscles are sore after intense exercise. What the very latest research seems to show about brain functioning is that brain cells have such a tough job of that they are *constantly* running in this overdrive mode just by being conscious. The only way to really clear out the toxins is for the brain to power down into sleep mode.

While we're awake, our brain cells accumulate various metabolic by-products such as the inhibitory neurotransmitter adenosine, which diminishes our mental focus. Recently, scientists in a National Institutes of Health-funded study used a new imaging device to look at the brains of mice while they were awake and asleep. They found that during sleep, some brain cells shrink, opening up the interstitial space between cells by about 60 percent so that cerebrospinal fluid can wash away neurotoxins and other by-products of brain cell function that accumulate while we are awake.[150]

An entire system of plumbing for this has only recently been discovered, in part because it nearly disappears while we are awake. This is the primary way that the brain clears away neurotoxins, and it works ten times better while we sleep than it does when we're awake. In addition to adenosine and other metabolites, this system has been shown to clear out beta-amyloid, a neurotoxin associated with Alzheimer's disease. One understanding of diseases like Alzheimer's is that it they are accompanied by an accumulation of beta-amyloid into plaques around brain cells, so it is quite possible that "rinsing away" the neurotoxins through more or better sleep could play a beneficial role.

So, one vital function of sleep is to help the brain clear out toxins. It detoxifies like an oil change for your car, and it has similar consequences for going too long between treatments.

What is the biological advantage of sleeping versus taking that time to continue to hunt, work, or wage war on sleeping rivals? At least part of the answer seems to be that sleeping is crucial to clearing away toxic molecules from our brains and also promoting brain plasticity so that when we are awake, we are much more capable of learning and thinking. These are functions that more than make up for whatever hours are lost to sleep.

How Much Sleep Do We Need?

Sleeping less than eight hours per night appears to trigger some powerful reactions in our bodies. Recent studies have found that getting just six hours of sleep per night for two weeks makes a person as impaired as someone who has gone for 24 hours without sleep.[151] How impaired is that? Another study found that going over 18 hours without sleep created the same level of cognitive and motor performance impairment as someone who is legally too drunk to drive, someone with a blood alcohol level of .10%.[152]

Getting six hours of sleep is clearly not enough. But what about seven? Researchers have looked at that, too. And while they find less impairment than in those who get six hours of sleep, even that extra hour isn't enough to let someone operate at optimum performance. According to one study, each day they get just seven hours of sleep per night, people become less and less able to perform a standard test of alertness and mental focus. This alertness level drops each day for three days until it stabilizes at a level lower than those who get eight hours of sleep per night.[153] So lack of sleep, even one hour less of sleep each night, has a measurable effect on our cognitive function, focus, and alertness.

According to recent studies by the National Sleep Foundation, Americans average 6.9 hours of sleep per night on weeknights. One study in Michigan found that of their random sampling, people got an average of 6.7 hours per night during the workweek and 7.4 hours per night on weekends.[154] This would mean that the people surveyed really *never* caught up on their sleep. They were chronically sleep deprived *on average*. Which means that for every person in the study who was getting the proper eight hours, someone else was severely deprived. However, after two weeks of sleep deprivation, the subjects of these studies report only being "slightly sleepy," regardless of the fact that their performance scores had dropped to their lowest levels during the study.[155] In other words, we are very poor judges of just how much our sleep deprivation is affecting our function.

Let There Be Light...And Dark

Our current level of sleep deprivation is a relatively new phenomenon for humans. It's a product of modern life that has rapidly accelerated over just the last few years as new technology has become commonplace. To understand some of these changes, let's look at how we used to sleep.

Nearly all living things on this planet evolved within a diurnal cycle, the 24-hour cycle of the earth spinning and exposing us to day and night. Plants and animals that adjust to this cycle are said to have a circadian rhythm. This means that the organism adjusts to changes in the light: sunrise, sunset, light, and darkness.

We naturally grow tired at night and wake in the morning. Before kerosene and then electric lights made it possible to see and work at any time day or night, our bodies were in perfect sync with the natural rhythm of the sun. The sun would rise. The light would flood us with hormones to tell us to get up and rev up our bodies and get ready to hunt prey, watch out for predators, and get things done until the lowering light levels of evening signal our bodies to start making hormones like melatonin to wind us down and prepare for sleep.

Melatonin is the main hormone responsible for helping us fall asleep. In addition to being a signaler, melatonin is also a powerful antioxidant that may have additional important roles in our health, so producing more melatonin is a very good thing if we want to stay healthy.

Have you ever experienced waking up on an extra-sunny morning after a good night's sleep and having the feeling like you can't wait to get going on the day? I grew up in Seattle where the winters were relatively long and gloomy, so when the summer mornings came, the slivers of sunlight sneaking in between the gaps in my curtains was enough to put me into a great go-get-'em mood. It was like some powerful stimulant was in the light itself that was impossible to resist. And in fact, there was. The specific wavelength of light in a sunrise triggers us to wake and get a move on, particularly if we've had sufficient sleep.

Throughout millions of years of evolutionary history, we saw a light day and a dark night in generally equal measure, depending on the season. At night we got tired and found a safe place to sleep. The idea of staying awake during the night would have been ridiculous, since a person could not see anything except perhaps on nights with a particularly bright moon. Humans would have been at a distinct disadvantage to animals that were adapted to nocturnal hunting. So our ancestors would find a safe place, conserve energy, and stay away from prowling animals. The theories about sleep providing these benefits weren't wrong. They just didn't tell the whole story.

When humans mastered fire, many things changed. Suddenly, our ancient ancestors could gather around the fire to stay warm, cook food, ward off predators, and socialize. The firelight had a nice orange glow, which does not interfere with melatonin production as much as the more-blue wavelengths of daylight that we see as a blue sky.

In the past 100 years since the invention of the electric light, all of this has changed. Along with the benefits of on-demand light when the world is dark, on-demand light has come as an enormous shock to our natural way of living, and sleep is what has suffered the most. The problem isn't just that we have more hours of light. It's also the kind of light. Today's fluorescent, LED, and other bulb technology offer "daylight," meaning bluish light, that signals our body not to produce melatonin and prepare for sleep. This is a benefit because it can keep you awake if you work all day in an office with little natural light. But it's not so great in your bedroom at the end of the day when you need to sleep.

By putting these technologies into screens like giant TVs or tablet computers held inches from our faces, we expose ourselves to very focused levels of daylight right up until a few minutes before we decide to go to sleep. No wonder we get so little sleep. We've created natural daylight and never really see the shift of colors at sunset or the lowering light levels of dusk. We sit with a tablet computer inches from our eyes until we switch it off and try to go to sleep. Only *then* do our bodies begin producing melatonin.

Dangers of Sleep Deprivation

When we don't get enough sleep, many changes occur in our bodies—none of them good. First, the brain does not have the ability to clear out the accumulated toxins, so it grows tired and less effective. The accumulated adenosine, an inhibitory neurotransmitter, fogs our thinking and our concentration, and focus suffers.

Other parts of our bodies also have profound adverse effects. Wound healing decreases. A study of rats found that those deprived of sleep did not recover from burns as quickly as those that got normal amounts of sleep.[156] In addition to slowing healing, we also become less able to ward off illness. Sleep has a big impact on fueling the immune system. Animals that sleep longer tend to have a higher white blood cell count on average.[157] **Studies on rats have shown that depriving them of sleep for just 24 hours reduces their white blood cell counts by 20%.**[160] In another study, rats kept from sleeping at all died within a couple of weeks.[159]

Certain kinds of sleep affect growth hormone levels. Slow wave sleep (SWS) has been shown to increase the amount of human growth hormone that men produce.[160] Although the question exists about whether a higher natural cycle of SWS causes higher growth hormone levels or whether a higher need for growth hormone pushes the body into SWS, it's clear that without enough sleep, the growth hormone does not get produced. Other hormone imbalances occur, especially those affecting eating. Inadequate sleep triggers our bodies to produce more of the signaling hormone ghrelin, which makes us feel hungrier. It causes us to produce less leptin, the signaling hormone that makes us feel full.[161] So our appetites get it at both ends, with more hunger and less satiety, making it very hard to resist overeating.

In a study published by the National Academy of Sciences, researchers in the UK subjected human test subjects to a week of sleep deprivation, about six hours per night, followed by a week of normal sleep. They discovered that sleep deprivation significantly alters gene expression of over 700 different genes.[162] Some genes are up-regulated, and others are down-regulated or made more or less active, respectively. This is breaking research, and the scientists are still looking into the specific changes due to this massive amount of changed gene regulation. But it's clear that getting insufficient sleep has a powerful effect on how our genes are expressed.

Lack of Sleep Can Make You Fat
With artificial light, especially our new daylight-type LEDs and fluorescents, we have clearly bypassed much of our bodies' evolutionary circuitry related to sleep and the circadian rhythm.

Before artificial light, the normal sleep cycle varied with the seasons. For any humans who lived outside the equatorial zones, when days were shorter in the winter, they responded by sleeping longer. Conversely, in the summer, they were up longer and slept less. The farther one moved from the equator, the greater this effect would be. Our bodies regulate the amounts of those key signaling triggers leptin and ghrelin we produce with shorter nights to make us eat more when days are long. What is the evolutionary or biological advantage of this?

I suspect that in summer, when food is plentiful and the days are short, our bodies use this short nighttime period to signal us to eat as much as possible and store that food as fat, because winter is coming. It was important that we do this, even if we had eaten all the food we needed that day. Our bodies needed to trick us into continuing to eat more food than we immediately needed so that we could store up energy.

In equatorial zones, where day and night are roughly equal, this has little effect, since the nighttime is the same year round. It's not necessary to store up a lot of resources for several months of cold and famine. However, in temperate, or even sub-arctic zones, the difference between day and night is increasingly more pronounced, as is the need to put on more winter fat to survive. So the farther we are from the equator, the longer our summer days will be, the shorter our summer sleep will become, and the greater will be our need to pack on the calories and store it as fat. This is so that we can survive, because the winters will also be more severe at these latitudes. At least that's how it's been for the past 100,000 years.

Today, by staying up late night after night with our faces shoved into lighted screens, we are tricking our bodies into thinking that we live in the longest-summer of all and that we desperately need to fatten up for the coming (harshest!) winter by eating as much as possible and storing it all as fat. And we do this year round. Is it any wonder that we find ourselves facing an epidemic of obesity? All our genetic programming is driving us to this. And we have digital devices to thank for it.

Sleep and Safety

Insufficient sleep is also an important public safety issue. Every year, numerous traffic accidents are caused due to drivers who are sleepy. The National Highway Traffic Safety Administration estimates that 100,000 accidents a year are directly attributable to driver fatigue. Various driving experiments have shown that sleep deprivation causes difficulty in driving, as measured in the ability to remain in the same lane of traffic. The results were similar to being legally drunk—ranging from a blood alcohol level of 0.07% to 0.10%.[163] Professional truck drivers who had been awake for 28 hours showed the same driving deficits as those with a blood alcohol content of 0.10%, legally drunk in any state.[164] Think of all the lives cut short or diminished because someone didn't get enough sleep and caused an accident.

At the extreme end, investigators have cited sleep deprivation as factors in the Three Mile Island nuclear accident, the meltdown of Chernobyl, the Space Shuttle *Challenger* disaster, and the *Exxon Valdez* oil spill.[165] That's an enormous cost for too little sleep.

Etcetera, Etcetera

The sleep loss and weight gain connection is clear, but insufficient sleep has also been found to contribute to numerous health problems including heart attack, heart failure, stroke, obesity, and several other conditions. Poor sleep has also been shown to increase blood pressure in young adults.[166] For people with hypertension, losing just half a night's sleep has been shown to increase blood pressure.[167]

As significant as the hard costs of insufficient sleep are, there's also an insidious effect that's difficult to tally—being tired leaves a person in grumpy and unpleasant to others and themselves. When you're constantly deprived of enough sleep, you just aren't any fun to be around, and that takes a toll on your happiness and that of those around you. Some research has shown that sleep deprivation's impact on mood is even more profound than its impact on cognitive function.[168]

The Benefits of Sleep

You can expect many benefits from getting eight hours of sleep every night. In addition to eliminating your drowsiness and improving mental focus through clearing out toxins at night, there are also many immediate and measurable benefits.

Growth, Learning and Brain Plasticity

Brain plasticity is the ability of the human brain to grow and change, developing new synapses and connections to deal with our changing environment and experience. It's learning new things.

Sleep, particularly rapid eye movement (REM) sleep, seems to be closely linked to brain plasticity. REM sleep and slow-wave sleep (SWS) play crucial functions in forming memories, particularly procedural memories, such as learning how to do something, and complex or emotionally charged declarative memory (facts).

Growing brains need sleep. This is especially true in childhood, when our brains grow faster than at any other time in our lives after gestation. Infants sleep 13-14 hours per day, with about half of that being REM sleep. Growing children also have high sleep requirements. But our brains to continue to grow and restructure themselves throughout our lives. And for that, they require sleep.

The REM sleep, where most dreams occur, is named for the rapid eye movement that occurs as we dream and process information in an almost real-time way. Some believe that this is a time similar to a computer defragmenting its hard drive, when our minds move memories from temporary storage to a more permanent form of memory. In the process, we reencounter some of these memories, learnings, and experiences as what we call dreams. In fact, REM sleep may be the portion that contributes the most to brain plasticity, new memories and learning.

In adults, REM sleep happens at different phases during the night, but they are not evenly dispersed. **Most REM sleep happens late in the sleep period. So if**

you are missing two hours of sleep per night, you may be missing out on *half* **of your proper amount of REM sleep.** Remember, this is the stage that's most critical to learning, new memories,[169] and possibly to fending off brain conditions like dementia and Alzheimer's disease.

Sleep More, Weigh Less

It doesn't sound right, but sleeping more can help you weigh less. Besides the obvious benefits of having more energy and desire to exercise when you are rested, there's strong evidence that not getting enough sleep triggers your body to put on body fat. Short sleep duration has been shown to increase the amount of ghrelin in our bodies. Remember that ghrelin is a hormone that our bodies make to tell us to feel hungry. Without ghrelin, we don't feel all that hungry, even if we need to eat. And with lots of ghrelin in our systems, we feel hunger, even when we have plenty of energy. So it is a very powerful part of our hunger response, and it looks like not getting eight hours of sleep a night makes our bodies create more of it. Amounts of sleep and ghrelin are inversely proportional, so less sleep contributes to weight gain and obesity.[170]

Whether it is because of the additional ghrelin, the reduced stress tolerance, or some other mechanism, sleep deprivation has been shown to make people more susceptible to hedonistic food stimuli like fast food ads and imagery.[171] People who haven't slept enough are more influenced by advertisements for food. Some researchers are concerned that America's chronic sleep deprivation may be one of the causes of America's obesity epidemic.

The National Health and Nutrition Examination Survey I (NHNES I) is a major study conducted by the Centers for Disease Control. It looked at over 8,000 people over the course of two years and then again three to five years later. The study found a conclusive link between low sleep and obesity, even controlling for other factors. Compared to people who slept seven to nine hours per night, people who reported sleeping just six hours per night were 27% more likely to be obese (not just overweight, but obese). Those who slept just five hours a night were 73% more likely to be obese.[172]

Not sleeping may be a more effective route to obesity than overeating, although they really go hand in hand. Real evidence shows that weight loss won't kick in until you start getting eight hours of sleep, seven nights a week.[173]

Sleep Is Sexier Than... Sex

A surprising finding shows just how sleep deprived we are, from a recent survey of 1,000 Americans. **The Better Sleep Council found that 61 percent of Americans and 79 percent of women would rather get a good night's sleep than have sex.**[174] If you ever needed a good reason to make sleep a priority for yourself and your mate, here it is. Add to the benefits of getting sufficient sleep feeling better, getting more done during the day, and having more fun at night. Suddenly, life is looking a whole lot better.

Show Me the Money!

If a better ability to manage your weight and more fun in the bedroom are not reasons enough to get more sleep, consider that losing sleep equates to losing dollars. Through lost productivity, lack of sleep is costing our country a remarkable amount of money. A study of employees at four U.S. corporations found that, compared to people found to get good sleep or have at-risk sleep habits, those with insomnia and insufficient sleep had significantly worse productivity, performance, and work safety outcomes. The study estimated fatigue-related productivity losses at $1,967 per employee per year.[175] Another study by the CDC found that over 40 million American workers, or about 30 percent of the work force, don't get enough sleep. As a result, they spend about eight and a half minutes of every hour distracted or in what's called *microsleep*, a state of momentary sleep people get when they're sleep deprived. **All of this adds up to over $63 billion a year in lost productivity.**[176]

No one has yet done a definitive study of exactly how much an hour per night of diminished sleep over a long period affects individual performance, but from my reading of the studies I've cited, I think it is safe to estimate at least a 25 percent reduction. That is, people who consistently sleep eight hours per night accomplish at least 25 percent more work in the same amount of time as the same person during a period of consistently getting just seven hours. If that's the case, then getting an additional hour of sleep to go from seven to eight hours effectively enables a person to do the equivalent of 10 hours of work during the day compared to their reduced net productivity of 7 1/2 hours. **The person who consistently gets eight hours of sleep is able to get *more than two extra hours-worth* of productivity from their day, while feeling better and being healthier.**[6] In some professions, such as mine, where quality is measured in terms of creativity, insight, problem solving, and articulation of ideas, the difference is even more dramatic. Remember, this is just the increased productivity for one additional hour of sleep per night. A person who consistently sleeps six hours per night or less would have an even more dramatic increase in productivity if they start getting eight hours of sleep per night. Still think that working late makes you more effective at your job?

So, lack of sleep makes you fatter, less sexy, less productive, more distracted, and grumpier, not to mention the many tangible ill effects it can have on your health. That doesn't sound like we're getting much net benefit for the extra hour or two of TV or Internet time we squeeze in each night at the expense of sleep, does it?

Supplement Support

Supplementation can help some of us drift off into restful, natural sleep, but supplements are not drugs. There are many pharmaceutical sleep remedies like Ambien that are designed to address America's sleep debt. Many of these are highly addictive and have dangerous side effects. And for most people, they are completely unnecessary if the patient would simply align his or her cycle to the natural circadian rhythms as described in this chapter. My advice: **Do not take pharmaceutical sleeping pills at all.**

A few natural remedies can support your body adjusting or readjusting to the natural sleep rhythms. One obvious and highly effective one is to simply take supplemental melatonin to make up for some of what our bodies do not make due to artificial light. I recommend taking a very small amount. Some evidence indicates that a little is good, but more is actually less effective and can lead to odd dreams, so I don't recommend taking more than 3 mg.[177] L-Theanine is a component of tea leaves that in purified from can improve relaxation and promote calmness, important before sleep. And finally, a supplement called 5-HTP (5-hydroxytryptophan) is a natural form of the amino acid tryptophan, which is a chemical precursor, and metabolic intermediate of melatonin and serotonin. 5-HTP is able to cross the blood-brain barrier and metabolize to melatonin to aid in drowsiness. In my own experience occasional use of all three of these in combination works well, without becoming habit-forming.

These supplements can be especially helpful in the first few days while traveling across time zones or adjusting to a new sleep pattern. Once your body has acclimated to the same bedtime and wake up time every day for a few weeks, supplements probably won't be necessary anymore.

PRESCRIPTION Nº4

1. Make an appointment

2. Lower the lights

3. Limit caffeine

4. Use the bedroom for two things

5. Sleep chemical free

6. Stay grounded

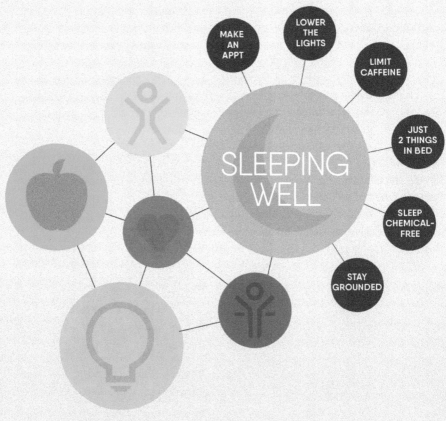

1. Make an Appointment

If you don't make the time to sleep eight hours each night, it simply won't happen. Most likely you already set your wake up time for each day, so simply count back eight hours and set your bedtime as well. It's simple math: if your alarm is set for 6 am and you still haven't gone to bed by midnight, well, you aren't going to get eight hours of sleep tonight, my friend. It sounds simple, but there's no getting around it. Most people schedule their wake up time but neglect to schedule when they will go to bed and turn off the light. This is a very simple adjustment but one you must make. Otherwise, you constantly risk falling into the trap of "one more thing to do."

So, give yourself a bedtime that is eight hours before your alarm clock is set to go off *and stick with your schedule*. This gives you the possibility of getting adequate sleep each night—without which, all the other actions you may take cannot possibly work.

If you're currently getting less than eight hours of sleep each night, it's natural that there will be an adjustment period. To ease the transition, some people recommend moving your bedtime 15 minutes earlier each day until it reaches the time you want. I don't think this is necessary, especially if you are particularly sleep-deprived. However, if changing your bedtime in smaller increments helps you, that's fine. I think you will adjust more quickly by making the adjustment once and perhaps supplementing with melatonin and 5-HTP during the first couple of weeks.

Now, while you're scheduling your bedtime, eight hours before your alarm is set to go off the next morning, I'm also going to encourage you to set it for the same time every day, weekdays and weekend.

I realize that some people may be tempted to throw the book across the room at this suggestion. You may be thinking, *"What? Give up sleeping in on weekends? That's the only way I'm making it!"* The classic way that most of us address our constant sleep deprivation is by sleeping a few extra hours on weekends. However, once you start getting adequate sleep *every night*, you will no longer need the extra sleep to catch up. So another benefit of regular, adequate sleep is that you don't waste prime weekend hours trying to catch up on your sleep from the workweek.

There's nothing "natural" about a five-day workweek. Our bodies have no mechanism for a certain schedule for five days and a completely different schedule for the other two. Just like animals, what our bodies seem to like best is consistency. Waking up later sets up a pattern of going to bed even later that night, which can become a viscous circle. Consistent sleep-wake cycles, on the other hand set up a virtuous circle where your body naturally knows when to wake and when to fall asleep, making both of them easier. You spend less time waiting to sleep at night and can get out of bed at your chosen time without feeling groggy or needing the snooze button. Once your body becomes used to a consistent sleep/wake pattern, you may not need an alarm clock at all.

The Snooze Button

I wish some things had never have been invented, like nuclear weapons or plastic water bottles. But the one that the most people probably use every day is the snooze button on their alarm clocks. Sure, it can feel great at the time—ten more minutes to doze. Unfortunately, it's a false solution. Once you alarm goes off the first time, your sleep cycle is disrupted, and the healthy benefits of sleep are over, no matter how many times you hit snooze.

Only your sleep deficit makes the snooze button seem like a good idea. When you're adequately rested, you'll wake ready to face the world. *So don't use the snooze!* If you have ten more minutes that you can afford to stay in bed in the morning, then set your alarm ten minutes later so you actually get the benefit of the extra sleep.

During the first few weeks of adjusting to your consistent daily eight-hour sleep period, you may be tempted to use the snooze button. My advice is to avoid the temptation. It gives you no real benefit and, in my experience, it will just delay your adjustment to this new schedule that will ultimately solve your sleep problems.

2. Lower the Lights

Our bodies need a certain adjustment period between day and night if we want to easily fall asleep. Even if you've set a regular eight hours for sleep each day, if you are bathed in the light of a computer, smartphone or TV until the moment you hop in bed, sleep will elude you while your body acclimates to the idea that the day is done.

To fall asleep, we need to promote melatonin production. Daylight signals our bodies that it is time to stay awake. Even small amounts will do this, so it's important to minimize these. It takes at least an hour of dim light for melatonin levels to begin to rise. Dimming your lights is very helpful since not only does it lower the level of the light in a room, but with incandescent bulbs, dimming also shifts the light toward the orange end of the spectrum. If you want to read and still be able to sleep, a reading light with a small incandescent bulb may still be a good solution. The thing you absolutely want to avoid is placing the backlit screen of a tablet or similar computer right up to your face where all that light completely halts melatonin production.

Once you go to sleep, your bedroom should be as dark as possible. Even the light from a small clock can interfere with melatonin production and reduce the quality of your sleep. If you can't completely darken your room, an eye mask to block all light can be extremely beneficial at increasing your quality of sleep.

Starting at least an hour before bed, but even earlier, if possible, lower the lights in your house. Turn off lights in rooms where you don't need them or put them on dimmer. Light chores like cleaning up the dishes are fine. Reading under a low light is excellent. This hour before bed should be a mini digital-detox. Avoid bright lights, TV and computer screens close to your face.

On my computer, I use a free program called F.Lux that matches the color spectrum of the screen to the outside natural light shades and Apple smartphones and tablets now have a brightness setting called "Night Shift" that eliminates much of the blue spectrum, both of which make a tremendous difference for me on those nights I have to work late and then try to get right to sleep.

3. Limit Caffeine
There's a lot of research to suggest that caffeinated beverages like coffee, tea, and *yerba maté* have many positive benefits for our bodies and that even the caffeine itself does us good. I'm not recommending cutting it out completely. However, *depending* on caffeine to get you through the day is a symptom of insufficient sleep. And having too much caffeine during the day, especially late in the day, can exacerbate sleep problems. If you wake up with the sun and *need* coffee to feel like you can function properly, that's probably an important sign that you are sleep deprived. But it will get better quickly as you get more sleep. Every person has their own caffeine threshold, but as a rule of thumb, stop having caffeine after lunchtime to make sleep easier.

Herbal tea is great and rooibos, peppermint, chamomile, and others can all be great afternoon or bedtime drinks. Remember, chocolate also has some caffeine, so don't overindulge in it just before bed.

4. Use the Bedroom for Two Things
Habits are extremely powerful drivers of behavior, and limiting your bedroom habits to two things, sleep and sex, can dramatically improve the quality of at least one. By reserving bed for these important things, when you go to bed, you'll be psychologically expecting to do one, or both, of these things. Our bodies' expectations are very powerful and help prime us for certain actions. If you read, work, or, worst of all, watch TV or use the computer in bed, you turn the bedroom from a sanctuary into a work and entertainment area and diminish your body's association between bed and sleep.

5. Sleep Chemical-Free
Almost all conventional mattresses off-gas numerous chemical compounds including formaldehyde, which you constantly inhale as you lay on the mattress.

Apart from keeping you awake and making you sleep poorly, this really isn't any good for you. By law in the U.S. and other countries, mattresses are required to have flame retardants, a requirement dating back to an era when many people smoked in bed. Most mattresses are then sprayed with brominated flame-retardant chemicals, many of which have known health and breathing hazards. All of these combine into a chemical miasma that you breathe all night long. If you sleep on a typical mattress, then the only good thing about being sleep deprived is at least you're spending a little less time breathing the harmful chemicals coming out of your mattress.

On a personal note, I will never forget the morning after my first night sleeping on an organic bed. I slept for nine uninterrupted hours for the first time since childhood. I awoke feeling as though I had been on vacation for a week. I was totally relaxed, and I was able to breathe deeper than I had in years. Since that day, I have slept deeply and fully on my organic mattress, and when I must travel the difference is profound. The morning after sleeping on an off-gassing chemical-laden mattress, I feel sick and groggy, even if I got "enough sleep."

An organic cotton mattress is a great option for sleeping well. First and most importantly, they are not sprayed with flame retardants or made with synthetic foams that leach formaldehyde. As a bonus, you're supporting a system of agriculture that considers its impact on the earth, and that's good for everyone. Natural latex mattresses are my favorite option for a great night's sleep. I sleep on a mattress by PranaSleep, which is 100% natural latex rubber and comes in a variety of firmness options. Flame suppression is required by law and is achieved through a mattress cover with non-offgassing fibers woven into it, so you can breathe and sleep like a baby. One warning, though. When looking for a rubber mattress insist on 100% natural rubber and beware the term "all natural", since this label means that it may be adulterated with up to 40 percent foam rubber. Note that if you buy a traditional mattress in the U.S., it must meet certain flame retardant standards which almost always means brominated chemicals.

A chemical-free mattress can be initially pricy, but they are ultimately well worth the cost for the long-term health benefits. If you cannot immediately switch to a chemical-free mattress, then wrap your mattress in a low density, food grade polyethylene cover, which will help seal in any chemicals that outgas from your current mattress. These are available online from a number of sources. While not as good of a long-term solution as a chemical-free mattress, this will significantly reduce your exposure and is very affordable.

6. Stay Grounded

Our bodies are receptive to electromagnetic frequencies and although the science is still new, I'm convinced that these frequencies can disrupt sleep just as light and sound can. Your brain is both a chemical and an electrical system, and outside

EMFs can subtly disrupt the electrical signaling required to rest and recover a healthy brain. Keeping cell phones off and other sources of electromagnetic fields (EMFs) far away from your body will lead to more restful and uninterrupted sleep.

Beyond minimizing stray EMFs, sleep can also be an opportunity to re-synch our body's frequency to that of the Earth. As I discussed in the Moving Well chapter, humans evolved to naturally synch our electrical current with that of the earth. Modern conveniences such as plastic or rubber-soled shoes and non-conductive building materials and elevated mattresses have broken this connection and electrical charges, stopping the flow of natural ions to quench damaging free radicals generated from our metabolism. But we can reconnect with the ground charge of the earth by sleeping on a mattress that connects us to this charge again through the grounding plug on every electrical outlet which literally connects to the earth. Since meeting the inventor Dr. Jeff Spencer several years ago and hearing how it had helped the U.S. Tour de France cycling team recovers from grueling workouts and ultimately win at the Olympic level, I sleep with an Earthing grounding sheet under my regular sheets. It makes a noticeable difference in both the quality of my sleep and almost eliminates the morning creakiness that I used to have (and still get after a night in a hotel bed).

HOSTING WELL

"We are more bug than human."

—*Dr. Deb Levy*

HOSTING WELL

HOSTING WELL

ere's a puzzler: What is *you* if most of the cells in your body are not you? No, that's not a zen koan, it's a remarkable way of looking at the nature of what a human body is actually made up of. You see, our bodies play host to perhaps *a hundred trillion* microbes in the form of bacteria, viruses, fungi, and simple animals. Amazingly, these microorganisms that live in and on our bodies actually outnumber our body's approximately 10 trillion cells by ten to one.[7] This sounds incredible and perhaps a bit disgusting on first blush, but there's no getting rid of all of these microbes. And you wouldn't want to if you could, because many of these organisms are absolutely vital for our health and well-being.

The Microbiome: Our Partners in Health

It seems that throughout our evolution—certainly since the first mammals and probably long before—microbes have been our symbiotic partners in survival. They have evolved right along with us to help us digest our food, extract additional nutrients, ward off illness, and even regulate our hormones. It's a win-win relationship: the microbes get a nice warm body to live in, one that walks around and finds food to eat. In exchange, the microbes help us extract energy and nutrients that would otherwise be unavailable to us. Many of these microbes actually create important nutrients that we need but cannot make for ourselves. Maybe just as importantly, they protect us from other microbes that would also try to colonize our bodies and wouldn't play so nice.

Let's face it: in nature, anywhere there is a nice warm place with a lot of food constantly moving through it *some* microbes are going to move in and set up shop. The beneficial microbes in our bodies have found a way to work with us and give back something useful. In exchange, our immune systems typically do not fight them off.

Our partnership with the beneficial microbes inside of us is proving to be more important than we initially realized, and new research is coming out constantly to reveal this crucial link. While we've long understood that microbes are important to our health, our scientific knowledge in this area is now exploding. The link between our health and our microbes has become so clear and compelling that some of the brightest minds in the world are now making it their life's work to learn more. So set aside your sensitivities for a moment, because this can get a little messy, but also remarkably fascinating, and the subject is crucial to our bodies' functioning properly. Let's take a good look at your microbiome—the microscopic ecology in and on our bodies—to see how it is vital for our good health.

Your Microbiome

It is likely that before you were born there were not any microbes on or in your body. In the womb, you receive nutrition through the umbilical cord and therefore don't have any digestion occurring to require or attract gut flora. All that changes at birth. When babies are born through normal vaginal childbirth, they are flooded with microbes from their mother's body that quickly colonize their skin and work their way into the infant's digestive system. Infants have been found to have their mother's intestinal flora in their upper gastrointestinal track within days of birth.[178] These are primarily *Lactobacillius and Bifidus* strains which help protect the infant from pathogens.

Babies born via normal birth are fully colonized by these *Lactobacillus* bacteria within the first month after birth. Babies born through C-section do not get these bacteria and are instead initially colonized primarily by *Staphylococcus* and other strains from their mother's skin. These babies can take up to six months to establish their normal intestinal flora.[179] Remarkably, a mother's body seems to alter its chemistry to favor certain bacteria prior to childbirth. In the third trimester, certain species of gut flora increase and others decline.[180] This seems to be the body's way of giving the new baby the right mix of microbes it will need to start out its life.

Gut flora goes through its biggest changes in the first three years but will continue changing throughout our lives for a variety of reasons. The biggest adjustments seem to happen right away as specific strains colonize our digestive systems. Breast milk is made up of about 20% human milk oligosaccharides (HMOs), which are special complex sugars that babies cannot digest. Why should a mother's body devote so much energy to creating an indigestible sugar? It seems wasteful. Well, this HMO is also called bifidus factor because it serves as a specific growth enhancer, or prebiotic, for *Bifidus* bacteria. The HMO helps one strain of bacteria, *Bifidobacterium longum*, to quickly overrun all the other bacteria in the gut to colonize the intestinal walls, effectively pushing out the potentially harmful bacteria.[181]

Breast-fed babies therefore, have a high proportion of *Bifidus* strains in their gut flora. Formula-fed infants have a wider variety of flora, but also more *E. coli* and *C. difficile,* which, under normal circumstances, are generally harmless but can be pathogenic. While researchers are still looking into this connection, it seems obvious to me that this is an example of evolutionary symbiosis. Human beings evolved to promote certain strains of beneficial bacteria within our guts—going so far as to alter body chemistry prior to birth to pass on select strains and then producing HMOs in breast milk to ensure that it would outpace other bacteria in the infant's gut. Likewise, *B. longum* evolved to take advantage of these growth factors and live harmoniously within our intestines. About 8% of the *B. longum* genome is devoted to HMO metabolism.[182]

Evidence exists that this intestinal flora is necessary for infants to develop the gut-associated lymphoid system,[183] the largest mass of lymphoid tissue in our bodies (roughly 80%). This is crucial for a proper immune system. In studies with newborn mice that had been kept sterile of these intestinal microbes, the mice were found to have underdeveloped intestinal immune systems.[184]

Definitions

Microbiome: The entire biome of microbes living in and on our bodies, both beneficial and pathogenic.

Gut flora: Microbes that inhabit the human digestive system, primarily the intestines. Often called Enteric bacteria.

Probiotic: Live microbes that inhabit the gut and benefit the host when consumed.

Prebiotic: Indigestible food components that feed beneficial microbes in the gut.

Synbiotic: A supplement that includes both probiotic organisms and prebiotic components.

After infancy, babies continue to acquire new bacteria. How do they do this? Well, you know how babies love to put things in their mouths, everything from hands to toys to dirt? That seems to be the primary way that new intestinal flora enter our bodies. Just a thought to make you feel slightly better when you see the dog lick your beautiful new baby's face or she sticks some dirt in her mouth. She's augmenting her microbiome! Of course, we get all kinds of bacteria this way, and only a small number become established in our gut. Fortunately, babies are surrounded by a variety of other humans and get a high proportion of human symbiotic bacteria from their families through touch.

By age three, when most children in Westernized countries are weaned and eating a wide variety of solid foods, our microbiome is largely in the form it will take for most of the adult life until old age.

Your Ecosystem
Our bodies create a wide variety of ecosystems for microorganisms to colonize. We focus on the gut flora because that is where the greatest amount of our microbes seem to be and because it has been studied the most. However, as science delves deeper into studying our microbiome, more discoveries will be made. And many are likely to be in areas outside our gut.

Our skin is our largest organ and it provides a vast area for bacteria and fungi to make their homes. Over 1,000 species of bacteria live on our skin alone,[185] and they vary greatly from our belly buttons to our nostrils to the spaces between our toes. As with our intestinal flora, some of these species appear to be beneficial and help protect us from colonization from pathogenic species. These harmful bacteria, like many *Streptococcus* and *Staphylococcus* species are also constantly present and prepared to take advantage of wounds.

Complicating matters, there are bacteria like *Pseudomonas aeruginosa* which can be beneficial in some circumstances and pathogenic in others. Normally, *Pseudomonas aeruginosa* creates antimicrobial compounds that kill pathogenic *Streptococcus* and *Staphylococcus* bacteria and many fungi including *Candida albicans*.[186] However, if the *Pseudomonas aeruginosa* enters the body, instead of just staying on the surface, it can cause a variety of infections. Similarly, gut bacteria can cause infections if they escape the intestines and enter the rest of the body, as can happen with a perforated intestine. However, on the whole, this bacteria seems to play an extremely important role in protecting us from pathogens. Removing *Pseudomonas aeruginosa* bacteria from our skin with topical or oral antibiotics can open us up to fungal skin infections.[187]

Our guts, mouths, lungs, ears, eyes, and genitals all have their own microbiomes. I think of our microbiome as being like a rainforest. Many different species are involved, and they are in constant competition for space and resources. Some of the species hurt the host, others help. The very vastness of the number of species plays a role in ensuring that no one species runs rampant and causes problems. We can take actions to make it easier for our beneficial species to thrive. Other actions, such as using antimicrobial chemicals in soaps, mouthwashes, and sanitizers, can indiscriminately wipe out wide swaths of our rainforest and create an opportunity for opportunistic and often pathogenic species to sweep in to take over that area. Because of this, I recommend staying away from anything anti-microbial unless you have an open wound or are going into the hospital for surgery. And yes, this includes mouthwash and hand sanitizers.

We typically discuss microbes using their scientific names of genus and species. This leads to a lot of foreign-sounding microbes that can be hard to keep straight sometimes. However, you are probably already familiar with many of these microbes by slightly different names.

Pathogens

Candida: This genus of yeast that lives on humans. Candida is responsible for "yeast infections," also called candidiasis.

Escherichia: This genus of bacteria is the "E" in *E. coli*, a species of bacteria that can cause virulent infections. *E. coli* are common in human gut flora.

Staphylococcus: This genus of bacteria live on the skin and respiratory tracts of many animals and also exist in the soil. Mostly they are not pathogenic, but they're also responsible for "Staph infections" of the skin and most dental cavities.

Streptococcus: This is a genus of bacteria that is responsible for "Strep throat," as well as many other infections such as meningitis, bacterial pneumonia, endocarditis an inflammation of the heart), erysipelas (a skin infection), and flesh eating necrotizing fasciitis. However, some non-pathogenic species of streptococcus are also among our microbiome, including one responsible for culturing yogurt.

Beneficial Microbes

Bifidobacterium: A genus of beneficial bacteria that makes up a large part of human gut flora. Also called *Bifidus* or formerly *lactobacillus bifidus*. You may recognize this from the ingredients list on your yogurt containers.

Lactobacillus: Another "yogurt bacteria" that is also responsible for sourdough, cheese, sauerkraut, kimchi, and many other fermented foods. This genus is also prevalent in the human microbiome. It is mostly beneficial, except that it is a bacteria responsible for some dental cavities.

Every Microbiome Is Unique

Every person's microbiome is unique, though it is highly influenced by those around you, especially those who were close to you in your first three years. Though we focus on the gut bacteria, because it's the largest component of our microbiome and also the one we know the best, we should remember that microbes are on every part of our body. Some areas, particularly orifices, host particularly heavy and often complex populations.

While there are hundreds of different species of gut flora, 30-40 species of bacteria seem to comprise about 99% of our intestinal flora. It appears that all human beings possess a small core of intestinal flora.[188] These have probably been with us since the dawn of man. Beyond these core microbes, there is quite a bit of variability from person to person and region to region. Some ethnic and regional groups may have very different gut flora, depending on the foods they eat and what their ancestors ate.

In 2012, researchers in France discovered that Japanese people host a unique form of *Bacteriodes plebius* that can digest porphyrin, a normally indigestible starch found in red seaweed, the kind used to make the sushi wrapper *nori*. The Japanese are the only people in the world who seem to have this unique gut bacteria.[189] The researchers postulate that when people first came to Japan around 40,000 years ago, they found themselves eating red seaweed as a significant new food source, and consequently, they also ingested various bacteria that lived on the seaweed and were able to break down porphyran. At some point, these ingested bacteria laterally passed this gene[8] to *B. plebius* and the gut bacteria acquired the ability to digest this starch. By making more food value available from red seaweed, the new strain of gut bacteria flourished in Japan and is now widespread there, although it does not exist anywhere else in the world.

To me, this is a fascinating incidence of non-human evolution benefiting humans, and a great example of the power of these microbes. No human genes changed or evolved in the seaweed example, and yet these humans benefited from the ability to get nutrients from an entirely different food source. Science may eventually discover numerous incidences of gut flora that are unique to specific populations. As we look at some of the things that our microbes do for us, from digesting foods to regulating hormones to creating vitamins and other nutrients, it may be hard not to think about other things. What could distributions of diseases or protective factors among certain populations turn out to be, in part, due to gut flora unique to those populations? With certain gut flora playing roles in obesity, depression, and other conditions, current research indicates that one day soon doctors may implant new strains of beneficial bacteria in order to ward off disease or improve health.

Beyond Yogurt

Of course, intestinal microflora has long been used to improve health. Most people's understanding of microflora starts and ends with yogurt. Yogurt is an ancient food present in numerous cultures around the world. Originally developed to preserve milk in the days before refrigeration, it appears to have been used medicinally to cure diarrhea since the 16th century and probably much longer.

Yogurt is traditionally milk fermented with a variety of bacteria. The manufacturers think it sounds more appealing to call them "cultures," but it means the same thing.

Some of these bacteria include *Lactobacillus* and *Bifidus* species and *Streptococcus thermophilus*. If these sound similar to some of the enteric bacteria that colonize our intestines during infancy, that's because they are. Supplementing with these probiotic yogurt bacteria can recharge our intestinal flora and push out harmful bacteria that may have taken up residence there. In the rainforest metaphor, eating yogurt and other probiotics is analogous to planting new seeds for the kinds of trees that we want to grow.

Yogurt typically contains just a few strains of probiotics, and they are usually listed on the package. However, our gut flora consists of around 500 strains[190] (some researchers believe the number is closer to 1,000[191]), and the majority of these strains cannot be cultured outside the body.[192] It seems that yogurt and a few other probiotics might help recharge a very small part of our microbiome, but just a part. We need to take good care of the rest of our gut flora because it is not as easily recharged. Furthermore, most yogurt does not contain a high enough level of probiotics to do much good and the typical yogurt cup is loaded with more sugar than a Twinkie so we need to look beyond yogurt for balancing the gut microbiome.

Clostribium difficile is a bacteria that naturally lives in our gut at low levels. It is notable because it is resistant to many antibiotics, a fast-growing weed in the rainforest. Imagine burning down a rainforest, but leaving one kind of weed that can easily survive the fire. With all the other trees and plants gone, this weed has ample room to spread and take over. This is essentially what can happen in your intestines when you take antibiotics. When you take systemic antibiotics, they knock out a good portion of your beneficial flora and *C. difficile* (also called *C. diff* or CDF) multiplies to take up all the available space in your intestines formerly colonized by more beneficial bacteria. If you've ever taken antibiotics and ended up with the runs, you've experienced *C. diff* in action.

In addition to antibiotic-associated diarrhea, *C. diff* is also responsible for more serious pseudomembranous colitis and the life-threatening condition toxic megacolon which can require the colon to be removed as a treatment. *C. diff* is becoming a problem in medical facilities where it can be spread rapidly, with fatal results.

To keep *C. diff* from becoming a problem, the easiest way to prevent it with the much more potent concentrations of probiotics found in supplements, which can help maintain the beneficial bacteria in the gut and keep the *C. diff* at its normal levels. Yogurt has been shown to help prevent antibiotic-associated diarrhea if taken while antibiotics are administered.[193] Once the *C. diff* becomes established, however, it appears that it may be too late for probiotics. Since *C. diff* is already resistant to many antibiotics it can be difficult to treat. Some antibiotics are effective against it, but increasingly, there are *C. diff* strains which defy them. In these cases, doctors need to turn to extreme measures to save patients infected with *C. difficile*.

Okay, hang on for a gross but fascinating part. The most effective treatment for *C. diff* that does not respond to antibiotics is to transplant stool from a healthy person into the patient overrun by *C. diff*. This can be done in several ways, from capsules to spray enemas. Like transplanting a big patch of rainforest, a cross section of a healthy person's gut flora is reintroduced to person whose flora is overrun by a pathogen. The result? This gut flora transplant cures 90% of cases,[194] usually where all other options have failed and the patient's life is in danger. And it typically starts to cure them within *hours*. Because it is so effective and often cheaper than antibiotics, many doctors are now considering this as the standard therapy for *C. diff* rather than a last resort.[195]

Remarkably, transplanting intestinal flora in this manner has also been shown to aid the symptoms of Parkinson's disease to the point where even neurologists could no longer detect its symptoms in some patients.[196] This is a very young science, but the research is exploding, and new discoveries are being announced all the time. This is suddenly a very hot area of research, because it offers so much potential. It seems that in the future we may see numerous treatments to unexpected ailments in the form of transplanting specific intestinal flora. Until then, we need to protect our rainforest and take good care of the gut bacteria that we have.

Benefits of Gut Bacteria

Let's take a look at some of the benefits we get from our microbiome—primarily our gut flora.

Disease Prevention and Treatment

It's not an accident that 80% our body's immune system resides in our intestines. The presence of gut bacteria seems to cause lymph tissue to grow, particularly during infancy. Our mouths and lungs have mechanical means to limit bacterial infection, but our intestines have to constantly swim in bacteria and so this area needs strong defenses. As the tale of the *C. diff* suggests, our beneficial bacteria are really our best defense against invading pathogens.

The gut flora and our immune cells interact in numerous and fascinating ways.[9] In short, the gut flora have various mechanisms to tell the body not to attack them, but to attack other pathogens instead. The gut flora plays important roles in directing the immune system's B- and T-cells that attack foreign bodies. They can also help shut off immune responses to compounds which have been ingested and spend time in the gut, which is one mechanism for reducing allergies.

Vitamins and Lipids

Arguably, our gut flora's primary job is to help us absorb nutrients that our bodies need. These microbes may also help us absorb water. They definitely aid in absorbing lipids, or fat molecules.[197] They also break down complex starches that we lack the proper enzymes to digest. A study of rodents that were raised to not have gut flora found that they needed to ingest about one-third more calories to maintain the same weight as similar rodents with gut flora. We don't know if the numbers are the same with humans, but clearly these microbes make animals more efficient at extracting nutrients from plant-based foods.

What is more important than the amount of additional calories we get is the form in which we receive them. Rather than simply creating simple sugars from these complex starches, gut flora turn them into short chain fatty acids (SCFAs) that are important to various bodily functions. Three of the main SCFAs are propionic acid (used by the liver to create ATP which powers all muscle motion); acetic acid (used in metabolism of carbohydrates and fats); and butyric acid. They play critical roles in the colon's immune response and may fight cancer, especially colon cancer.[198]

These SCFAs also aid in metabolizing and absorbing other nutrients such as B vitamins, vitamin K, biotin, and sterols.[199] Some gut flora also seem to be able to break down certain carcinogens, like those from charred meat.[200] These naturally occurring carcinogens can lead to breast and colon cancer, so fostering the bacteria that metabolize them could be of significant benefit to their hosts. This sounds important, as most everyone eats grilled meat. What do we take?

Weight Management
With the additional calories and fats that our gut flora help us digest and absorb, you'd think that they would be making us fatter. In actuality, the reverse seems to be true: a healthy microbiome can regulate body weight and help us stay at a healthy weight.

In one experiment, mice were given low levels of antibiotics while very young to suppress the proper formation of their gut bacteria. Within six weeks, these mice gained 10-15 percent more fat mass than those that did not receive the antibiotics.[201] The mice with the suppressed gut flora got a lot fatter, possibly in a similar way that farm animals gain weight when put on antibiotic feed.

Sadly, another study suggests that this plays a role in human development as well. In a study published in Nature, over 10,000 human babies who received antibiotics within the first six months of life were later tracked and found to have a 22% increased chance of being overweight.[202] But couldn't this just be from too much TV and video games? Apparently not. Although exercise is important, a longitudinal study of overweight and obese children in Plymouth, England, found that physical inactivity is the result, not the cause of obesity in children.[203] Could having failed to establish a proper gut flora due to some combination of C-section birth, bottle feeding, early antibiotics, and a dietary or environmental antagonists be contributing to childhood obesity? And if so, are these children doomed to be overweight all their lives or could something be done about this?

This leads me to one of the most astounding studies I've read in a long time, one that challenged my own assumptions about being overweight. In a study published in *Science* in late 2013, researchers harvested the gut flora of human twins where one twin was overweight and the other was not, and then transplanted it into mice. The mice that got the normal weight twin's flora were unaffected, *but the ones that receive the microflora from the overweight twin soon became overweight*[204]. To me this is very clear evidence that our intestinal flora plays a role in causing obesity.

However, if getting the wrong set of bacteria only made a person obese, this would be a troubling report. Fortunately, the same study offered some very promising news. It seems that when the researchers introduced the lean twin's gut flora to the now overweight mice that had received the other twins' flora, the new lean microbiome can take over, *if the mouse is fed a low-fat diet that's high in fruits and vegetables*. The opposite, however, is not true. The lean mice don't get fat if the overweight twin's flora is introduced.

What's happening here? It would appear that **certain microbes aid in leanness**. The overweight twin's flora is missing these microbes so the mice get fat. When the new leanness-promoting flora are introduced, they face a gut already colonized, but they can prevail if the right diet exists in the host. On the other hand, the mice that initially get the leanness-promoting flora are fully established and so introducing new flora don't have any effect. In other words, there seem to only be leanness-promoting flora. **Obesity is promoted when these flora are missing, rather than being the product of some strain of obesity-promoting bacteria**.

Another mouse study examined specific strains associated with being slim, and found a greater prevalence of a type of gut bacteria called *Christensenella minuta was not only associated with slimmer, leaner mice*, but that reduced weight gain could be transferred when *Christensenella minuta* was transplanted into a germ-free mice.[205]

The science of gut bacteria and human health is evolving from animal research to human research at a rapid rate. In humans, two particularly important probiotic cultures are the *Bifidobacterium* and *Lactobacillus* families, because they are both associated with a healthy and balanced digestive tract. But new insights into the way colonies of these microorganisms interact is revealing new insights every month.[206] I find it increasingly likely that we'll one day have gut flora transplants as a cure for a number of conditions—especially obesity.[207] Until that day, it is important to take care of the gut flora we have and eat a diet rich in foods that will protect and help our intestinal flora.

Mood and Hormones

Our intestinal flora seem to have the ability to influence our mood and mental state by releasing certain chemical substances. For example, in studies, when humans and rats have been supplemented with probiotics *Lactobacillus helveticus* and *Bifidobacterium longum* they have shown less anxiety and fewer stress markers, such as lower serum cortisol, when put in challenging tests than those without the probiotics.[208] The mechanism is not yet well understood. However, certain bacteria clearly have the ability to modify human mood. One soil-born bacteria, *Mycobacterium vaccae* has been shown to release chemicals that have anti-depressant effects on people who come in contact with it, usually through gardening, by stimulating serotonin and norepinephrine production in the brain.[209] So if these bacteria have this ability, it's very reasonable to believe that those bacteria that evolved along with us have similar capabilities.

Supplement Support

Probiotic, prebiotic, or symbiotic supplements can be highly beneficial. Symbiotic supplements have both probiotic and prebiotic components. In a healthy body, gut microbes outnumber human cells ten to one. If you are actively protecting your microbiome from germ-killing biocides (called "preservatives" in the food industry) like BHA, benzoates and chlorine, and regularly eating a variety of fermented foods and prebiotic rich foods, then supplements may not do you much more good.

There are specific times when I am sure to supplement with probiotics (I get plenty of prebiotic fibers in my regular diet.) First, I take probiotics any time I have been on antibiotics. I also like to rev up my immune system with fresh probiotics at the start of cold and flu season each year. The human gut microbiome is one of the most exciting and popular areas of scientific research at present, and our insights are growing by the day. One of these insights is that probiotics work in colonies in the gut, so I supplement with a multi-strain rainforest ecology rather than some single "hero" strain. Look for a probiotic with at least 10 strains that have been proven to be beneficial. The colony forming unit (CFU) rating of the supplement should be in above 50 billion and an enteric coating, which protects the capsule through the acid of the stomach so it will dissolve in the intestines. It will help maximize the amount of live cultures that reach the gut. I rotate my probiotic purchases between brands with the idea that each company delivers a different mix of strains and variety of clinically supported probiotic strains provides for a healthier gut ecology.

PRESCRIPTION №5

1. Don't Kill Your Partners

2. Cut The Chlorine

3. Ditch The Antibacterial Soap

4. Choose Living Foods

5. Feed Your Microbes

6. Use Antibiotics Only When
   Absolutely Necessary

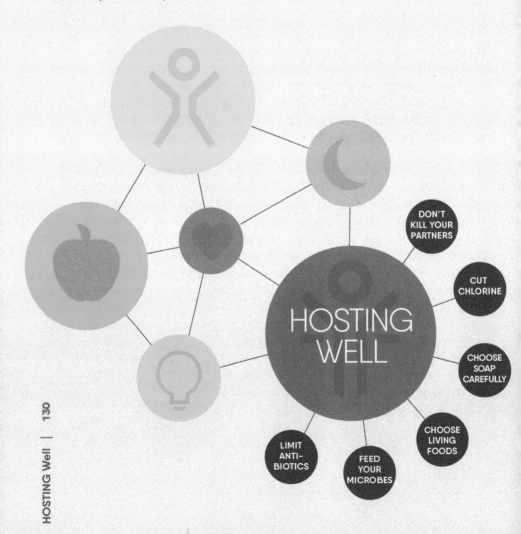

HOSTING WELL

DON'T KILL YOUR PARTNERS

CUT CHLORINE

CHOOSE SOAP CAREFULLY

CHOOSE LIVING FOODS

FEED YOUR MICROBES

LIMIT ANTI-BIOTICS

I find the discoveries in the area of the human microbiome to be absolutely fascinating. We are at a unique time in history, when new discoveries in this field are coming out with great regularity. These microbes—most of which co-evolved with their human hosts—may contain 100 times more genetic material than we do ourselves. This topic is rapidly expanding how we think of our own genetics and evolution. I cannot wait to see what science discovers next in this arena.

Although the science of the human microbiome is comparatively young, there are some clear lessons here about how we should help preserve these important partners in health. I believe that the lack of information is all the more reason to tread very cautiously where our microbiome is concerned. It is not at all hard to believe that future discoveries may prove that our gut flora plays a significant role in obesity, diabetes, cardiovascular disease, cancer and even mental disorders. What then can we do to preserve our rainforest of beneficial microbes so that they can protect us?

1. Don't Kill Your Partners
Clearly, the very first thing we can do to protect our microbiome is to not indiscriminately kill it. Unfortunately, modern life is awash in chemical compounds that are made to do exactly that. With the best of intentions, we have flooded our water with chlorine, a broad spectrum anti-microbial, added anti-microbial compounds to products that don't really need them such as dish soap and mouthwash, and included chemical preservatives that kill all kinds of microbial life and persist for exceedingly long periods within our bodies.

2. Cut the Chlorine
Chlorine is a broad spectrum antimicrobial agent used to purify water. Every public drinking water system in the U.S. is mandated to use chlorine. There are, of course, some distinct benefits to this—namely that it kills bad bacteria so we don't get outbreaks of cholera or *E. coli* overcoming large populations.

However, once we drink the chlorine or bathe in it, it can work to kill the bacteria in and on our bodies. We don't yet know how significant the impact is on our microbiome. Most likely, some bacteria are more sensitive than others. There's a chance that important strains of our flora are disproportionately knocked out by chlorine from our drinking water. Filtering the water you drink and bathe in can remove chlorine and help preserve your beneficial microbes. Filtering shower water is particularly important not only because it protects our beneficial skin microbes, but also because the warm water of the shower means that we inhale this chlorine too, which could affect the microbiome of our lungs. Studies have shown that we could get 50-90% of our daily chlorine exposure from showers[210] and that long hot showers lead to even greater exposure.[211] So if you want to enjoy a hot shower, it's wise to filter the chlorine from the water.

Filtering chlorine from the water coming into your house is the best solution, but it can have a high upfront cost. Placing chlorine filters on showers, refrigerators, and faucets also works just as well, although you do need to replace these periodically. Filter pitchers such as those made by Brita are another good option for getting the chlorine out of drinking water.

3. Ditch the Antibacterial Soap

Antibacterial soaps have taken the modern world by storm to the point where in many places it's hard to find soaps that *don't* contain these chemicals. Remarkably, these soaps have been found to be no more effective that regular soap in killing pathogenic bacteria. In fact, washing with plain soap is also effective against viruses, which antibacterial soap is not. So antibacterial soaps don't do anything to prevent the common cold or influenza. The FDA is currently reexamining the supposed benefits of antibacterial soaps.[212]

The primary chemical in these soaps is triclosan, a chlorinated aromatic chemical which kills most bacteria and fungi. Triclosan can be converted to dioxins in water, particularly chlorinated water, and it tends to persist and accumulate in the body. Triclosan has also been shown to be an endocrine disruptor. I have many concerns about the use of products containing triclosan, because it may accumulate in the body and kill important beneficial organisms. It almost certainly kills beneficial bacteria on our skin, leaving us open to pathogens. Because it does not seem to be any more effective than plain soap and water or maybe more dangerous, I avoid antibacterial soaps wherever I can.

Triclosan is also used in mouthwashes and toothpastes, which I find to be even worse than the soaps. You swish triclosan around in your mouth, swallowing a little, and wiping out a chunk of the rainforest. It's not well understood how long triclosan persists in the body, but it seems to last quite a while and spread far and wide. Triclosan has been found in human breast milk,[213] where it has no business being. It has been shown to be an endocrine disruptor in animals,[214] so numerous reasons exist to avoid it, beyond the havoc it plays on our microbiome.

4. Choose Living Foods

Since our microbiomes are clearly of importance to our health, it's natural to want to help it function. Adding more beneficial microbes is a great place to start—like constantly planting new seeds in our rainforests. What foods can you eat to help your gut flora keep you healthy? These living foods provide live probiotics with every bite:

Yogurt, Kefir, and Cheese

Yogurt is a great place to start. It's commonly available and is often fortified with a number of beneficial strains, mostly *Lactobacillus bulgaricus* and *Streptococcus thermophillus*. However, many yogurts are not as beneficial as they should be.

Many yogurts on the market are so loaded with sugars that they are essentially junk food. To get the greatest benefit from yogurt, look for organic plain yogurt with "live and active cultures." Even better is to make your own yogurt at home with organic milk. Homemade yogurt has far more beneficial bacteria than commercial yogurt, and because the fermentation recently occurred these probiotics are in a more active state.

Goat milk yogurt is my favorite. The fat molecule in goat milk is smaller and easier to digest than the fat in cow's milk. And goat milk, the most widely consumed dairy milk on the planet, does not contain the pro-inflammatory A1 casein protein found in most cow's milk. I find it digests better, and I feel and perform better after a delicious bowl of goat milk yogurt with chia seeds and blueberries.

Kefir is a similar product to yogurt. It's made by adding kefir grains—a culture of symbiotic lactic bacteria and yeasts—to goat, sheep, or cow's milk. Kefir is more acidic than most yogurt and has a slightly different probiotic makeup. Many soft cheeses like goat cheese also have live cultures. Aged hard cheeses typically have fewer surviving probiotics than softer cheeses.

Sauerkraut, Kimchi, Pickles, and Miso
Sauerkraut is made of thinly sliced cabbage and a lot of salt. It goes through a fermentation process with lactic bacteria. Kimchi is a similar dish usually made from cabbage, although many kinds of kimchi exist. This is combined with garlic, chili powder, and often other vegetables. Many pickled vegetables made with brine undergo a similar fermentation process. When these foods are not sterilized or cooked[10], the lactic bacteria are probiotics that have been shown to include a wide variety of species.[215]

A study published in 2011 looked at several overweight and obese subjects who ate either fermented or unfermented kimchi daily for four weeks. Those who ate the fermented kimchi were found to not only slim down and improve their waist-to-hip ratios, but also improve their fasting glucose levels and cholesterol levels.[216] So while kimchi includes a lot of fiber, vitamins, and phytonutrients, the probiotics of the fermented kimchi seem to play a key role.

Miso is another food that contains live cultures. Miso paste and soy sauce are the products of a fermentation of barley, soy, and wheat. The soy sauce rises to the top, the miso sinks to the bottom. Natural miso, like that used to make Japanese miso soup, has *lactobacillus acidophilus*.

5. Feed Your Microbes
While getting a variety of probiotics is important, feeding the microbes you already have may be even more crucial. Remember, most of our gut flora cannot be cultured outside the body, so the probiotics we get represent only a small—but

important—cross-section of out beneficial bacteria. While we can't easily replenish those other bacteria by eating live cultures, we can eat foods that encourage them to flourish.

These foods that help feed our beneficial gut flora are called prebiotics and they mostly consist of complex carbohydrates that we cannot digest on our own. Some prebiotic foods include onions and garlic, asparagus, whole grains, and bananas. The pectin in fruits and jams are also prebiotics. A few food additives, especially fibers, like inulin (from Jerusalem artichokes), psyllium seed husk (a bulk fiber), and acacia gum are important prebiotics. As researchers discover more about our gut flora, they are likely to discover more foods that act as prebiotics as well.

Prebiotics are important food and activators for your gut bacteria. Some strains of these bacteria likely lie dormant (or as spores) until their specific foodstuffs arrive in our intestines. By consuming complex carbohydrates that feed the gut flora, you activate them and encourage them to grow.

Some fermented foods are not probiotic but are still prebiotic. Red wine does not transfer any beneficial gut flora that we know of but its polyphenols still seems to be prebiotic for *Bifidus* bacteria.[217] Similarly, apple cider vinegar that many people drink for the purported health benefits is not probiotic but the apple pectin is prebiotic.

6. Use Antibiotics Only When Absolutely Necessary

Antibiotics are a modern medical miracle. I'm extremely grateful that my family lives in a time and place when we have access to modern antibiotics. They save lives and I do not want to demonize them. That said, antibiotics have been overprescribed in America and other countries and that is causing numerous problems. The problem we hear about the most is the emergence of antibiotic-resistant strains of formerly controlled diseases. But perhaps equally important is the damage done to our microbiome when taking courses of systemic antibiotics.

Taking systemic, broad spectrum antibiotics is essentially like burning down your rainforest to try to kill a weed. There are times when they are necessary. Only take antibiotics when they are absolutely necessary and take locals if appropriate. And please, never take antibiotics for a cold or other viral infection where the antibiotics cannot help. Some people have pressured their health care providers to prescribe them even though they would do no good. Doctors are less inclined to honor these requests today, but I expect it still happens. However, when a doctor prescribes antibiotics, ask if there is a more targeted form that is appropriate. It's also a great idea to increase your probiotic and prebiotics—either from food or supplements—while you are on antibiotics to preserve as much of your beneficial flora as possible.

STAYING WELL

"He who has health has hope,
and he who has hope has everything."

—*Arab Proverb*

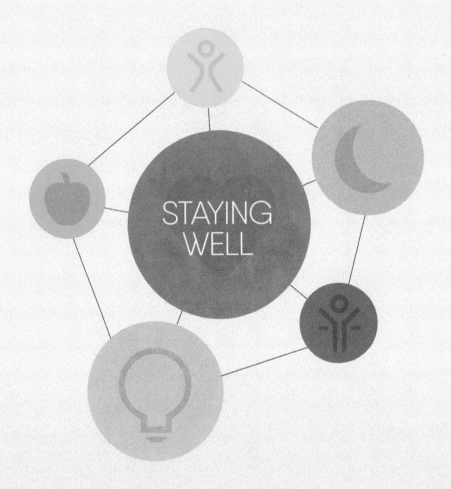

STAYING
WELL

STAYING WELL

Most of the time, we think about being "well" as avoiding colds and the flu so we can go about our daily schedule. We eat right, get some sleep, try not to drink too much, and generally keep healthy so we don't miss a lot of work or feel lousy. That is the working definition of staying well for a lot of people.

For some people, however, staying well has an entirely different meaning. To those who battle ongoing diseases like MS, cancer, lupus, multiple chemical sensitivity, chronic fatigue syndrome, and other conditions, staying well can mean the difference between a productive life and one spent as a prisoner to their disease.

I have lived with multiple chemical sensitivities for years. It made me change my career, my lifestyle and even my geography. Even now I must avoid flare-ups by carefully managing my environment and what I put into my body. Staying well is what allows us to live a productive life. All the healthy choices I make about diet, exercise, sleep, my microbiome, and the rest do me very little good if I allow myself to get sick. So here I want to talk about what you can do to stay well.

What Makes Us Sick?

Our bodies are remarkably good at taking care of themselves. Why then, do we get sick at all? We get sick when our bodies' defenses are overrun. It's my belief that the key to staying well is to work both ends of this equation: to minimize exposure to pathogens and environmental chemicals that can make us sick and also to keep our defenses strong through adequate sleep, exercise, a health-promoting diet, and practices that preserve our beneficial microbiome. I'm not a doctor, but when I look at people who are sick, it often appears to me that not only was there exposure to the disease, but there was a simultaneous lowering of the defenses that let the illness take hold.

Throughout this book I've been discussing good practices for promoting robust health: getting eight hours of sleep each night and setting regular daily schedules; exercising and avoiding sedentary behavior; seeking out healthy foods and avoiding empty calories and additives; and protecting and fostering the beneficial microbes that play an integral role in our good health. Following the Living Well Program will give anyone an excellent foundation in warding off illness. But there's a missing piece for today's world if you want to avoid illness—avoiding the invisible threats.

Surrounded by Invisible Threats

The modern world can be a dangerous place. We rarely have to worry about large predator attacks or uncontrolled famines as our ancient ancestors did, but we are surrounded with dangers that they could never imagine—in fact, most of these dangers cannot even be seen. Our food is commonly laced with additives that are known to be carcinogenic. Objects we handle every day include compounds that disrupt our hormones. Pathogenic, and increasingly antibiotic-resistant, bacteria and viruses abound, often in places like hospitals where we go to get well, not even more ill. While we seek to improve our general health through the steps we've discussed elsewhere in the book, we need new guidelines to keep these invisible threats from affecting our lives.

The chemicals and germs that we encounter daily can have disastrous effects on our health. Infectious diseases are bouncing back to new levels of virulence after decades of largely being pushed back by advances in vaccines, antibiotics and other treatments. Industrial and agricultural chemicals are often found to be harmful only after having been in widespread use for years. For example, a 2014 report conducted by the Harvard School of Public Health and published in *Lancet Neurology* found that a growing number of chemicals are linked to brain disorders in children. The report found new evidence about six newly recognized neurotoxicants that have negative health effects on children: manganese, chlorpyrifos and DDT (pesticides), tetrachloroethylene (a solvent), and the polybrominated diphenyl ethers (flame retardants).[218] The report's authors warn that many more chemicals likely remain unidentified as neurotoxicants. Of course, these chemicals were harmful all along but are only now understood to be so. How many more chemicals that we encounter daily are harming our health? To me the answer is to minimize contact with these chemicals as much as possible.

Protecting Your Castle

Dr. Ignaz Semmelweis was thought insane by his colleagues in 1847 when he suggested the radical idea that if doctors would wash their hands after dissecting cadavers and before they went to deliver babies, they might reduce the high levels of Childbed Fever that his Vienna clinic was experiencing[11]. In the century and a half since then, we have not come up with many ideas that are simpler or more effective for eliminating contaminating our bodies than simply washing our hands.

In interacting with the world, we constantly pick up not only germs but also chemical residues. Washing our hands frequently with soap and water and avoiding touching our eyes, nose and mouth where these invisible threats can actually enter our bodies creates a create a clean zone around our bodies so that less gets in. This powerful "first line of defense" is one of the best ways to protect ourselves from getting sick. In fact, simple hand washing can prevent about 30%

of diarrhea-related illnesses and about 20% of respiratory infections (such as colds).[219]

Remove Your Shoes

Taking things one step further, there is a very simple habit you can create that will eliminate an enormous amount of pathogens, pesticides, and heavy metals from entering your living space: simply take off your shoes when you step inside your house.

A large study done in Salinas, CA, found widespread traces of agricultural and other pesticides in the dust of private homes.[220] A similar study found that toxic coal tar— a suspected carcinogen—is tracked into homes from streets and driveways.[221] The answer to both of these problems is to remove the shoes at the door. This is a common custom in many homes around the world. When we walk, we pick up all kinds of bacteria from the soil, animal feces, and garbage. In 1991, the EPA released a study referred to as "The Doormat Study" which found that home where the occupants used doormats and removed their shoes at the door reduced the amount of lead dust and other chemicals in the home by about 60%.[222]

Dr. Charles Gerba, a researcher well known for his studies of microbe transmission performed an unpublished study for the Rockport company about the potential benefits of washable shoes. He discovered that the shoes he tested averaged 421,000 bacterial units per square centimeter, including *E. coli* and other bacteria known to cause human infections.[223] By contrast, toilet seats have been found to have only about 1,000 bacterial units per square centimeter. **The bottom of your shoes have several hundred times more bacteria than your toilet seat.**

Dr. Gerba's study also looked at how well these bacteria transferred onto floor surfaces and found there was a transmission rate of 90-95%. And this study just tested for bacteria, not environmental pollutants, as the others did.

Removing shoes at the door keeps all these bacteria and pollutants in a small area near the entry. In Japan, it's traditional to leave outdoor shoes in a small alcove and switch to slippers within the house. Slippers are commonly provided for visitors. This is a great practice to adopt in your own life. You'll keep your home free of more toxins and probably have to spend less time cleaning as well.

Carpets and rugs tend to accumulate more of these pollutants than hard surfaces, meaning that this is even more important for homes that have carpets. Pets and young children spend a lot of time at floor level getting greater exposure to these pollutants. Walking over the carpets also kicks the dried pollutants up into the air as dust, which can be inhaled.

For me, the first line of defense in keeping pollutants and pathogens out of my body is to keep them out of my living space. Take off your outdoor shoes when you get home and leave them away from your primary living area. Wash your hands when you arrive home from anywhere. Wash your hands frequently throughout the day after touching anything potentially dirty or well handled by others. Keep your hands out of your mouth, eyes, and nose—the easiest entryways into your body for these invisible threats.

Our hands are the gateways to our bodies. In daily life as we touch things, we pick up viruses, bacteria, and chemical residues. Most people know to wash their hands after going to the bathroom, but **depending on where you've been, you may want to wash your hands *before* you go to the bathroom**.

Obesogens: Avoiding Xenoestrogens, BPA and Other Endocrine Disruptors

An important invisible threat to minimize in our lives is estrogen-like compounds. These can come from natural sources, like soy and other plant compounds or from synthetic chemicals. These chemicals are called "obesogens", because they can chemically influence our bodies to become obese.

Estrogen is a sex hormone found in humans and other mammals. Both males and females generally have both estrogen (the female sex hormone) and testosterone (the male sex hormone) although they typically have very different levels based on gender. Our bodies typically regulate the amount of sex hormone quite efficiently. However, this changes when estrogen-like chemicals (also called xenoestrogens meaning "foreign estrogens") enter our bodies.

Because xenoestrogens closely mimic estrogen in the body and because estrogen controls numerous actions, exposure to these xenoestrogens can have a powerful effect on our bodies, particularly in disrupting the endocrine (hormone) system. It has been implicated as a cause of the early onset of puberty in girls. In 1950, the average age for the onset of puberty in girls was 13.1 years. In 2010, it had dropped to 10.5 years—according to new research from Germany.[224]

In women, elevated estrogen levels has been linked to breast, cervical, and endometrial cancers. In men exposure to these compounds may lead to testicular cancer, infertility, and malformed testes in young males.[225] It may also reduce male testosterone levels. Most xenoestrogens are considered endocrine disruptors meaning that they interfere with the normal function of human hormones, including causing weight gain and obesity.[226] The research around exposure to xenoestrogens is still growing, but so far everything seems to point to the common sense reaction that exposing our bodies to fake hormones does not do us any favors.

Sources of Obesogenic Xenoestrogens

One of the more troubling realities of xenoestrogens is just how prevalent they have become. The one that most people are familiar with is soy. Soy is a bean that has been a traditional food crop in Asia. In the U.S. it is grown as a wide-scale agricultural crop in rotation with corn to improve future corn yields. Because much is grown and used largely as animal feed, agribusinesses have spent a lot of money trying to create marketable soy products. One of those products is soy isoflavones—also called soy phytoestrogens. These plant-based estrogen compounds have been shown to reduce the symptoms of women going through menopause[227] as well as some other purported benefits.

Research, however, has cast doubt on the health benefits of soy. An August 2005 report from the DHHS Agency for Healthcare Research and Quality, found that there was no substantial evidence that soy protein or soy isoflavones provided any benefit in the previously claimed areas of bone health, cancer, reproductive health, or neurocognitive function.[228] However, animal studies have shown that soy isoflavones can cause breast cancer.[229] In human studies, women who supplemented with soy protein were found to have proliferation of epithelial cell in the breast.[230][231] These types of cells are the most likely to become cancerous. Some of the research on soy is conflicting, however. Some studies have shown that women who eat soy may actually receive a protective effect against breast cancer.[232]

Avoid Obesogens: Become BPA-Free

Naturally occurring phytoestrogens seem less harmful than synthetic estrogens. Bisphenol-A (BPA) is a chemical added to plastics such as water bottles and also used as a lining for some metal cans. By law, all aluminum cans must be coated to prevent the food from contacting the aluminum directly, and the industry standard coating contains BPA. BPA is an endocrine disruptor and "obesogen" (a chemical that makes people fat) that increases both the number of fat cells a person has and the size of those cells.[233] As an obesogen, BPA in beer can linings may be a contributing factor to the familiar middle-aged "beer belly". However, it's BPA's ability to cause illness that is most troubling.

BPA is highly regulated in Canada, though not in the U.S. Studies have found that people with high levels of BPA in their urine were significantly associated with heart disease, diabetes, and abnormal liver enzyme levels.[234] The study, published in the *Journal of the American Medical Association* in 2008 recommended that the U.S. follow Canada's lead in tightly regulating BPA's use.

Studies have associated BPA with altered hormone levels[235] and decreased sexual function in men,[236] recurrent miscarriages in women,[237] and decreased immune function in people under age 18.[238] It has also been associated with increased incidence of brain tumors[239] in human studies and cancers[240] and neurological issues[241] in animal studies.

A study released in 2012 had the very disturbing finding that the neurological effects of BPA are passed down for at least four generations in mice.[242] It remains to be seen whether this applies to humans or to BPA's other negative effects, but it seems entirely reasonable based on this research that **ingesting BPA now could have negative effects for your great grandchildren and beyond.**

So, BPA is bad enough when it is used in hard plastics that leach into the contents of water bottles or from the linings of aluminum cans or tomato sauce cans. However, a story published in *Science News* reported that perhaps the biggest exposure that most people have to BPA is from store receipts.[243] Most credit card and grocery store receipts are made by spraying a loose coating of powdery BPA and ink onto paper. When this paper is pressed or heated, the BPA and ink bind and appear on the paper. However, the rest of the BPA remains loose and powdery on the receipt. It can be absorbed through the skin, but it is almost certainly picked up on the fingers to be easily transferred to other parts of the body or any food that you handle without first washing your hands. A single receipt can have hundreds of times more BPA than a person could get from drinking from a BPA-laden water bottle. And for those people who handle receipts as part of their work, the exposure could be remarkable. I recommend not touching store receipts. Skip the receipt, have it emailed, or just snap a photo with your cell phone instead. If you do touch a receipt, wash your hands immediately and don't touch your face or food until you do so. If you work in a job where you must handle receipts, wear gloves.

Phthalates are another type of endocrine disruptor used in plastics production. While not technically a synthetic estrogen, phthalates still disrupt human hormone function in similar ways. A cross-sectional study of men in the U.S. found that those with the highest levels of phthalate metabolites were strongly correlated to insulin resistance and obesity.[244] They also seem to have marked effect on male endocrine systems and have been called "anti-androgens." Specifically, they seem to reduce some physical and behavioral markers of masculinity in males whose mothers are exposed to phthalates in the womb.[245] They also seem to contribute to breast cancer in women[246] and asthma in children.[247]

Eliminate phthalates
Phthalates, another class of obesogens, are used to soften plastics, particularly PVC type plastics. They are uses in numerous products from flooring to baby toys to erasers, and even medical devices such as catheters. Most soft plastics are made that way by including phthalates in the plastic—the softer they are, the more phthalates they likely contain. Because of the way that phthalates are bound into plastics (they are just held in place, not chemically bound), they are released quite

easily into the environment. They are also absorbed not only through breathing and ingestion but also through skin contact.[248]

Both BPA and phthalates are common plastic additives that have been shown to be endocrine disruptors that can easily leach out of plastic containers. While there is growing awareness about these chemicals among the public and progress in better regulating them, the invisible threat to our health continues. **New research is showing that *nearly all* plastic products release compounds with estrogenic activity—even if they are labeled BPA-free.**

A 2011 study published in *Environmental Health Perspectives* independently sampled a wide variety of plastic products and found that nearly all leached chemicals having detectable estrogenic activity. This included baby bottles and chemicals specifically labeled as BPA-free. The study concluded that many plastics are being labeled as free of estrogenic activity because they are only sampled with one type of solvent rather than using testing that more closely mimics real-world use.[249]

My recommendations here are simple. Don't drink from plastic water bottles, and don't buy tomato products in cans unless they're labeled BPA-free. It's also best to avoid plastic containers when eating or reheating food.

BPA, phthalates and other synthetic estrogens and endocrine disruptors are rampant in our environment—particularly our indoor environments. I feel that these are going to be found to be even more harmful as this research continues. You can reduce your exposure in the following ways:

- Do not drink beverages from soft plastic bottles.
- Do not buy tomato products in cans unless they are labeled BPA-free.
- Avoid soft plastics, particularly with food. Wash your hands well after handling soft plastics.
- Infants and women who are pregnant or trying to become pregnant should avoid all plastic products possible.
- Avoid handling thermal paper receipts

Eat Organic and Skip the Pesticides

Modern agriculture uses a wide variety of pesticides, fungicides, herbicides insecticides, and other chemical sprays. It should come as no surprise that since these are chemicals that have been created as poisons to kill animals, plants, and microbes, that there's a good chance that they don't do a lot of good in our own bodies. These chemicals have, for the most part, gone through testing and an EPA approval process. However, EPA-approved pesticides such as DDT, toxaphen, alderin and others have later been found to be harmful and banned, so it's reasonable to expect that this is likely to happen again. Further, some sprays that are not licensed in the U.S. are still used in other countries to grow food that ultimately arrives here for consumption.

One way that pesticides and pollutants enter your home is on your shoes or hands. However, we regularly bring these chemicals into our homes (and later our bodies) on our food. Conventionally raised fruits and vegetables are literally coated with insecticides, fungicide, herbicides, fertilizers and other agricultural chemicals. In fact, these chemicals have usually been mixed with spray adjuvants called "stickers" that help them stick to the plants and stay there longer through watering and rainfall. Rinsing these chemicals off fruit in the sink difficult due to these stickers. Many pesticides are also systemic—meaning that they are absorbed into the plant itself. There's no way to fully rinse off a systemic pesticide so the best bet is to choose organically grown fruits and vegetables as discussed next.

I am highly suspect about the safety of consuming pesticides. Apart from the direct long term affects, I am also concerned about how these biocides will affect the human microbiome. Research on the importance of our beneficial flora is only beginning and research on the long term safety of eating pesticides is scant—particularly on the pesticide cocktails that we may regulary consume from a broad diet rich in fruits and vegetables. To me this is one area where not enough research has been done yet and until we know a lot more, it does not seem safe to roll the dice.

Because pesticides and other agricultural chemicals can be difficult or impossible to fully remove by rinsing, the best way to avoid them is to buy organic food whenever possible.

Organic foods are produced without chemical fertilizers or synthetic sprays. Because they aren't pumped up with these chemicals, the yields are often lower and the farming is often more labor intensive. For this reason, organic food is typically more expensive than "conventionally grown"[12] foods. However, because organic foods have been found to contain much lower pesticide residue and more vitamins and phytonutrients[250][251], I think the extra money is well spent.

I've been buying primarily organic produce for the past decade and since then I've seen two important trends emerging. First, it is much easier to find organic foods— both in more mainstream supermarkets in many parts of the country, and in a growing number of specialty markets. So it's easier to find organic foods and they're now available in more variety and options than before.

The second trend I've noticed is that the price premium on organic food has been dropping as it has moved from a niche product to a more mainstream one. Organic food does still come at a premium over conventional, but the price difference seems to be dropping.

In the past, I advocated always buying organic versions of the so-called "Dirty Dozen" produce foods with the worst amounts of pesticides published each year by the Environmental Working Group (EWG). These included foods like apples, peaches, spinach, and potatoes because they were either heavily sprayed or had skins that you eat, therefore increasing the amount of pesticides you'd get.

There is now a complementary list of foods from the EWG called the "Clean 15" that are supposedly safer to buy as conventionally grown crops. This list, also from the environmental Working Group, includes things like cantaloupe, grapefruit, and avocados. Items on the "Clean 15" list need to have fewer than 4 types of detectable pesticides—while many had none. This sounds great until you understand that these tests were taken after the foods were washed and peeled. Almost all foods on the "Clean 15" list have thick peels that were removed before testing. So these are not foods that actually have fewer pesticides, they just get peeled off before testing.

One big concern I have about the "Clean 15" is that they have just as many pesticides; they just get washed and peeled before testing. I understand the EWG's goals in shining a light on the types of foods that people should definitely be eating organic because there's no peeling a blueberry. However, I am concerned about buying foods like cantaloupes—a very heavily sprayed crop—under the idea that it's a low-pesticide option. After all, you will still handle it, set it on the counter, place it near other fruit, and generally cross-contaminate your kitchen with pesticides.

I now believe it's important to buy all produce and dairy organic to reduce the amounts of pesticides and other chemicals that we bring into our homes and put in our bodies.

Avoid Toxic Metals

Certain toxic metals (often referred to as heavy metals even though not all heavy metals are toxic and not all toxic metals are heavy metals) can pose health hazards. These include lead, mercury, cadmium, arsenic, radioactive metals and excessive amounts of some common metals like copper. Like pesticides and pathogens, the best way to avoid these is to keep them out of your home and to minimize outside exposure.

Toxic metals can be particularly dangerous because they tend to accumulate in our bodies and break down very little if at all. Most of the research done on toxic metals has been in the hazardous effects that they have on developing fetuses and young children. However, there are really no accepted safe levels of exposure to these metals and I believe that further research will show that they have just as insidious effect on adults—although these effects may so far be harder to detect and directly attribute to toxic metals. Science is about what can be proven and sometimes these associations between health problems and toxic metals exposure are difficult to prove. Maintaining good health, on the other hand is about making good choices based on available data—you don't need conclusive proof to make an informed choice to stay away from toxic metals and pesticides even if they have not yet been conclusively proven to cause specific illnesses.

The toxic metals most commonly encountered include mercury, lead, arsenic, and cadmium.

Arsenic

Arsenic is found in the natural environment in some abundance in the Earth's crust and in small quantities in rock, soil, water and air. About one third of the arsenic in the atmosphere comes from natural sources, like volcanoes and the rest comes from man-made sources like treated wood, pesticides and coal burning.

Arsenic is a well-known poison implicated in several famous poisonings throughout history including Napoleon and Simón Bolívar. It shortens the lives of cells and reduces their energy by inhibiting cellular enzymes.

Industrial processes such as mining, smelting and coal-fired power plants all contribute to the presence of arsenic in our air, water and soil. Environmental contamination also occurs because it is used in agricultural pesticides and in chemicals for timber preservation. However, the most common source of arsenic poisoning is well water and the easiest way to avoid this is to have your well tested periodically. The controversial oil-drilling method called fracking (hydraulic fracturing) seems to increase the amount of arsenic in groundwater, so if you live in an area where this type of oil production occurs, test more frequently.

Arsenic is also a common component in many pesticides, so reducing pesticide exposure will also reduce your exposure to arsenic. Commercially raised chicken also has arsenic from a feed additive that helps keep the meat pink in the butcher's case.[252]

Cadmium

Like arsenic, cadmium is found naturally in the environment and is released through mining and smelting. It, too, enters the food chain from uptake by plants from contaminated soil or water. Cadmium is extremely toxic and even small amounts can have powerful effects on the body including irreversible kidney damage and death from inhalation. Cigarettes and industrial fumes are major sources of cadmium—and cadmium has been found to accumulate in the soil and water around industrial environments. In fact, China is facing a serious cadmium problem at the moment because it has used industrial wastewater containing cadmium to irrigate crop fields in its "rice bowl" district of Guangzhou—one of its main rice growing regions but also a thriving industrial zone. In 2013 the Chinese government encountered an uproar when they announced that nearly half the rice they tested from Guangzhou fields was contaminated with high levels of cadmium. This problem may be much bigger than the test results revealed, as the Chinese government may be loathe to announce the full results in the future following the uproar from the Guangzhou district.[253]

Another source of cadmium exposure in humans can be from shellfish. Shellfish like oysters are filter feeders and pick up toxins from their environment. Oysters farmed in areas with high levels of cadmium can absorb the element. However, one study has shown that there is low bioavailability of this cadmium in human consumption, possibly because of the high amounts of zinc in oysters.[254] (Our bodies prefer to take in zinc when available and one way to keep cadmium absorption low is to eat foods with plenty of zinc.)

Lead
Lead is a well-known toxic metal that is known to affect childhood development.[255] In adults, it can have a variety of symptoms that are often difficult to diagnose because they can be subtle and vary based on exposure means and levels.

Luckily, lead continues to be removed from paints, toys, and gasoline (except aviation fuel). Currently the greatest risk of lead exposure is the paint from old buildings and from industrial complexes. Lead is a good example of how we can significantly reduce exposure with regulation and reformulation—even though the pollution that is already released into the environment can never be fully removed.

Mercury
Mercury is a remarkable metal for many reasons. It is one of just two metals that are liquid in temperatures humans can tolerate. It has numerous chemical uses. And of course, it is both highly toxic and easily absorbed through the skin.

Our greatest source of mercury exposure is from eating fish—particularly fish from high on the marine food chain. Mercury enters the atmosphere from the burning of coal (and from volcanoes). It precipitates into the ocean and fresh water with rain and is absorbed by small marine creatures. As big fish eat smaller fish they accumulate the small amounts of mercury that they had absorbed. The effect is magnified as fish move higher up the food chain. Large fish-eating fish such as swordfish, shark, king mackerel, grouper and tuna have high levels of mercury. Eating these more than once or twice a month could lead to accumulating mercury in your body.

We can also be exposed to mercury through vaccinations. A compound called thiomersal, which is used in the preparation of some vaccines such as flu shots, contains small amounts of lead. It has largely been phased out of production since 1999, but do ask about it when receiving vaccinations and insist on thiomersal-free (also called "preservative free") preparations. There's no point injecting any amount of mercury into your body if you can avoid it. For other vaccines, request a new vial and ask that they shake it to evenly distribute any preservatives to avoid getting an outsize dose of preservative due to settling.

Get Your Shots

For most of human history, people lived in small family or tribal groups that were not large enough to spawn virulent infectious diseases. Humans needed to settle into cities before populations were large and dense enough to support such diseases.

Most infectious diseases that humans contract have emerged as mutations from animal diseases. Diseases tend to be very selective about what animals they can infect—most have only a few hosts. However, diseases often mutate or take on the lateral transmission of genes. So when animals live in close proximity with humans, from time to time a mutation in the disease allows them to "jump the species" to humans—and a new human disease arises. This happened in 542 A.D. when a disease of rats living in newly crowded cities caused the first wave of bubonic plague, and it is true today when poultry workers in densely populated Asian poultry farms are contracting new strains of bird flu.

Infectious diseases are a product of living in densely packed populations and in close contact (for some) with animals. It's a relatively modern problem and we are all extremely fortunate to live in a time where there is a modern solution: vaccinations.

Vaccines are made using several different processes. They may contain live viruses that have been attenuated (weakened or altered so as not to cause illness); inactivated or killed organisms or viruses; or inactivated toxins (for bacterial diseases where toxins generated by the bacteria, and not the bacteria themselves, cause illness). To your body, it is as if you had the disease because the immune system knows how to make the antibodies to fight off these viruses as they attempt to infect you (provided the virus has not mutated enough that the antibodies no longer recognize it, which happens fairly rapidly with influenza).

The inventors of various vaccinations—Edward Jenner, Louis Pasteur, Jonas Salk, Thomas Francis, Jr. and many others—were heralded as great heroes when they created new vaccines to protect against an illness. When Jonas Salk announced on the radio that his polio vaccination was safe and effective, the nation celebrated within minutes. Amazing, as this was before Twitter. Salk was soon brought to the White House for a Rose Garden ceremony, where President Eisenhower awarded him a presidential citation designating him "a benefactor of mankind." New York City offered Salk a ticker-tape parade, which he declined, and the U.S. Congress essentially invented a new award to present him, the Congressional Medal for Distinguished Civilian Service, among countless other awards and honors. Today, however, in the poster-child for all "rich country problems" people in developed nations fret about the safety of vaccinations for themselves and their children based on faulty, discredited research and miniscule numbers of people who experience side effects.

The Vaccination Controversy

After decades of protection from vaccines, it is now fashionable to question them. In 1998, Andrew Wakefield, then British surgeon and medical researcher had a paper published in the respected medical journal *The Lancet* a respected medical journal. This paper linked the measles, mumps and rubella (MMR) vaccination with autism and inflammatory bowel disease. The study was later thoroughly discredited as fraudulent and retracted by *The Lancet* in 2010.[256] A reporter looking into the original study found falsified data and called it an "elaborate fraud."[257] Andrew Wakefield was suspected of having a profit motive in performing lucrative tests for litigation against vaccine companies.[258]

Though scientists had begun doubting Wakefield's findings and many of his coauthors had retracted their part of the publication in 2004[259], the damage was done. Vocal support from celebrity Jenny McCarthy (whose medical research qualifications include Playmate of the Year and appearing in *Scream 3*) brought this issue to the tabloids, *The Oprah Winfrey Show*, *Larry King Live*, and other venues encouraging people to avoid vaccinations, even after Wakefield had been thoroughly discredited.[260]

And indeed, during this time there were some large jury awards to parents of vaccinated children even though public health officials believe they were unfounded and some vaccine makers halted production until shield laws were passed to protect them.[261] In the UK, MMR vaccination rates dropped from 92% to 80% in just two years,[262] and Japan stopped requiring MMR among childhood vaccinations. Today, Japan is considered a "measles exporter" by the CDC.[263] With the drop in vaccinations, measles, mumps, and rubella have increased, and people have been sickened and injured for life by these preventable diseases.

Vaccination is both a personal and a public health issue. If only one person were to choose to not have an immunization, he would only be putting himself at risk of the disease—and that risk would be quite low given all the other people who were vaccinated. However, as more people choose to avoid immunization, they put others at risk as well because they increase the chances of transmission. A person who chooses not to receive a vaccine may contract the disease and recover but still transmit it to another person who does not. Today, even though the MMR-autism connection has been roundly discredited, the controversy persists in the minds of many that there is "something wrong" with vaccines.

No vaccination controversy exists in the medical community, where there is a clear consensus that vaccinations do not cause autism. I am concerned about vaccines that include thimerosal (most vaccines in the U.S. do not) because of the mercury exposure, but I do not think they cause autism. There's no evidence for this. If you have children, make sure that they get their vaccinations – just insist that they use a new vial and shake it prior to administration. It is a chance to prevent terrible, life-threatening diseases. After all, it is very hard for you to be living well while your kids are sick.

Flu Shots

Influenza is the infectious disease that we all know well. Each winter it comes around again to re-infect you, even if you've had the flu many times before. That's because there are multiple strains of the virus, and they mutate rather easily—even passing around genes as they move between humans, birds, and mammal hosts.

A study published in the journal *Vaccine* calculated the annual cost of influenza at $25.7 billion ($10.4 billion in direct medical costs, $16.3 billion in lost earnings).[264] The drug store Walgreens performed a Flu Impact Survey of 1,200 nationally representative Americans and found that U.S. adults missed 230 million work days and U.S. children missed 90 million school days to influenza in the 2011-12 flu season.[265] Aside from the normal seasonal flu, there have been three flu pandemics in the last century responsible for millions of deaths. Researchers expect more pandemics in the future.

Each year, the WHO Global Influenza Surveillance Network publishes it's assessment of the strains it expects most likely to be prevalent in the following winter season. Three strains are prepared (in 2013 some vaccinations included four strains) over the course of several months. For people who receive these vaccines, it is as if they have had the flu three (or four) times in terms of gained immunity.

The flu vaccine is highly effective, however, people sometimes doubt its efficacy for three reasons. First, the strains that the WHO recommends are an educated guess that must be made many months in advance and sometimes an unexpected strain becomes more prevalent. Additionally, people often feel like they have the flu when in fact they have a "flu-like" illness or "stomach flu" (gastroenteritis). Finally, it takes about ten days to acquire immunity from the vaccination. People can catch the flu during this period and feel like the vaccine didn't work.

The CDC recommends annual flu vaccines for children up to 5; anyone over 50; pregnant women; and anyone with a suppressed immune system or chronic lung or cardiovascular disease—among others. I believe it is worthwhile for everyone to get a flu shot every year (provided there are adequate supplies of vaccine—which there usually are). It builds up immunity to influenza without the suffering and lost time of actually getting the disease. It's one of those things were everyone wins. I opt for the preservative-free version, which is available by request. For the cost of about $30 (probably paid by your insurance) it helps reduce the severity of the flu season for all of us, saving money, time and pain of actually getting the disease. For me, it's a lot easier to stick with a work, sleep, and exercise schedule when I'm not sick as a dog with the flu.

Maximizing Immunity

When you get vaccinated, research has shown two things you can do to maximize your immunity. The first is exercise. Two studies have shown that exercising on the day you get your flu shot can give you up to double the immune protection from the shot (measured in the number of antibodies you produce). The procedures tested included either lifting moderate weights for 20 minutes with the arm the shot would be given a few hours *before* the vaccination[266], or doing 90 minutes of moderate cardiovascular exercise *immediately after* the shot.[267] Both procedures seem to double immunity. So get a workout before or after your shot to increase the benefits of vaccination.

While exercise increases the immunity gained from vaccines, pain relievers lower it. A study in 2006 found that taking ibuprofen or other common non-steroidal anti-inflammatory drugs (NSAIDs) such as aspirin, Tylenol, and naproxen *reduced* the immunity one would gain from the vaccine.[268] Interestingly, it seems that inflammation is a crucial part of the immunization process. (The weight lifting before getting the shot most likely promotes additional immunity by creating localized inflammation in the arm muscles where the shot will be given.) So, when you get any vaccine, it's best not to have pain relievers for a week after the vaccination. Ibuprofen and pain-relieving doses of aspirin seem to reduce immunity the most. Very low doses of aspirin—like those used to prevent heart attack and stroke—have less effect. I would recommend avoiding all NSAIDs for a week after getting a vaccine. If you're on a low-dose aspirin regimen, talk to your doctor about this.

Cleanse Your Body from the Inside

Cleansing diets and fasts have been popular for years. Many current versions include a fast, some kind of "miracle fruit" extract, and perhaps some fiber and (hopefully) lots of water. There are so many versions of how to cleanse. Most claim that toxins build up in our bodies and that going for a few days eating only cabbage soup or drinking water with lemon juice and hot peppers will help you naturally shed them. The problem is that none of them are very effective.

As part of the research for this book, I looked for any studies that supported the concept of removing the "toxins" that these Detox Diets promote and I couldn't find any. The truth is that our bodies cleanse themselves continuously. This is mostly done through the liver and kidneys, which filter out toxins (quite effectively) and our intestines. By fasting, you actually slow down the passage of food in your intestines and reduce its normal cleansing function. These fasts do not lead to sustained weight loss success and may even train your body to hang on to fat when you go back to more normal eating.

You can detoxify your body by following the Living Well Diet. If you feel the need to cleanse, then do it naturally. Focus on high-fiber fruits and vegetables, fermented foods, and cruciferous vegetables (broccoli, kale, etc.). Drink lots of water, get lots of sleep, and rest your digestive system by fasting 10-12 hours per day. Keep your liver healthy with the right nutrients, so it can do its job every day. You just don't need any more cleansing than that.

Other cleansing plans such as exotic enemas, foot pads, potent laxatives, prolonged starvation or "juice-only" programs are similarly without basis and may cause harm through dehydration or other means.[269]

Supplement Support

Most readers will not need any supplements for healthy detoxification, since with the clean fuel and reduced toxic burden from the Living Well Diet your body will do an effective job of cleansing on its own. However, for people with multiple chemical sensitivities (like me) or others with occupational exposure to chemicals, excessive alcohol use or conditions that require more rapid clearing of toxins or xenoestrogens it is extra critical to keep the liver supplied with the vital components to enable it to do it's job of continuous detoxification.

Your liver is an amazing organ that plays a critical role in health, detoxifying metabolic wastes, hormones, and environmental toxins in a 3-phase process. Phase 2 is a critical stage where toxins are neutralized or literally detoxified, and this process relies on a combination of key micronutrients and enzymes. I take a combination of supplements (for which I have a patent pending) to ensure ample substrates to allow proper Phase 2 detoxification of environmental pollutants that are unavoidable in daily life. These include a broccoli seed extract rich in sulphoraphane and indole-3-carbinol, two components from brassica vegetables that provide a source of the crucial Phase 2 liver enzyme glutathione S-transferase (GST). GST requires ample amounts of the co-factor glutathione so my supplement also includes N-Acetylcysteine (NAC)—a compound that replenishes liver glutathione to ensure that Phase 2 detoxification can continue. To promote the elimination of toxins via the Phase 2 liver detoxification pathway, I also include 1,000 mg of Calcium D-Glucarate, a compound found in apples and other fruits that inhibits the beta-glucuronidase enzyme to help insure that molecules the body has chosen for excretion are metabolized and ready for removal from the body rather than being recirculated.

This combination of supplements has made an enormous difference in my daily health and ability to function at a high energy level, engage in business (and pleasure) travel, and survive the inevitable exposures that used to take me out of the game for days or weeks.

The other supplement I take daily is 250 mg of an extract from the cell walls of baker's yeast called Primuna®. This is the patented and clinically studied form of beta glucans. Beta glucans are a special type of dietary super fiber found naturally in foods like oats, barley and yeast. Primuna uses a specific form, beta 1,3/1,6 glucans derived from the cell wall of a highly purified, proprietary strain of baker's yeast *(Saccharomyces cerevisiae)* that activates key immune cells that safely enhance immune system. Over $300 million in research has been spent on the platform behind this extract so far to develop a version of it as a pharmaceutical drug. In supplement form, Primuna® primes the most prevalent cells in your immune system, called "neutrophils". Neutrophils are the front line of your immune defenses, patrolling your body looking for foreign invaders such as viruses and bacteria and killing them before they can multiply and overwhelm the host (that's you). By priming neutrophils and making them more vigilant, this yeast extract helps keep the body healthy. Neutrophils have about a 5-day life in the body, and once primed by Primuna, they stay primed for their entire cellular life.

PRESCRIPTION №6

1. Leave the Outside Out

2. Avoid Synthetic Estrogens

3. Skip the Sprays

4. Eat Low on the Food Chain and as Organic as Possible

5. Filter Your Water

6. Maximize Your Immunity

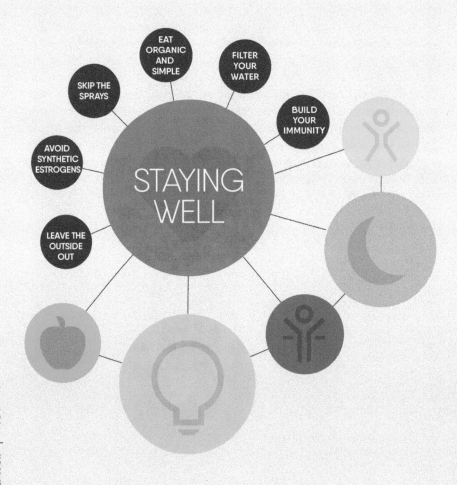

Staying Well is the last Pillar of the Living Well Program. It is the key to protecting the good health and habits you've built throughout the other Pillars. Here's my prescription for staying well:

1. Leave the Outside Out
Washing your hands and leaving your shoes at the door are simple but powerful habits for keeping your home safe from whatever you might have been exposed to outside. Keeping the outside out of both home and body have measureable and clinically validated benefits for health. And walking around barefoot has the side benefit of keeping you grounded.

2. Avoid Synthetic Estrogens
Plastics are an inescapable part of the modern world, but that doesn't mean you have to eat them. Keeping plastic containers out of the microwave, choosing filtered water in a glass over bottled water, and insisting on a ceramic or stainless steel coffee mug instead of Styrofoam can dramatically cut your exposure to the synthetic estrogens in plastic. Avoiding skin contact with thermal paper receipts or washing your hands thoroughly after touching them can also significantly reduce this common source of synthetic estrogens that can wreak havoc with your body's natural hormonal systems.

3. Skip the Sprays
According to the EPA, indoor air quality is two to five time more polluted than outdoor air, on average. Those household chemicals that you have to lock up from children are hazardous to your health. Collectively, we dump 32 million pounds of toxic chemicals down our drains each day, just from household cleaning chemicals. That doesn't count what goes into our indoor air. Since we spend more than 80 percent of our time inside our homes and offices, which are increasingly well-sealed for energy efficiency, poor interior air quality is a serious problem. Sprays contain anti-microbial chemicals that can have a detrimental effect on your health. As a general rule, if you can spray it into the air from a can, it's probably bad for you. For me, the rule is don't breathe in the same building where anything has been sprayed.

4. Eat Low on the Food Chain and as Organic as Possible
Big fish eat little fish, and little fish eat tiny fish, and tiny fish eat plankton. In general, the larger and longer-lived the animal, the greater the toxic load of that animal. A 20-year-old swordfish has many times the level of environmental pollutants as a four-month-old sardine. So, to minimize the negatives, eating low on the food chain only makes sense. Unless you are a vegetarian, I recommend making animal protein— whether it's fish, meat, poultry or dairy products—an occasional part of your diet rather than the "main event" of the meal in order to help reduce your overall chemical load and to reduce the load on the planet.
Eating low and organic helps keep agricultural chemicals out of your body, since these chemicals tend to concentrate in animal fats and the most toxic versions are not used at all in organic agriculture.

5. Filter Your Water

Our bodies are 60% water, and water is one of the highest-volume and most controllable inputs into our bodies each day. Filtering your tap water to remove chlorine and fluoride provides pure, clean, great-tasting drinking water at a fraction of the cost or environmental impact of expensive and wasteful bottled water, and without the plastic. A Brita or equivalent pitcher and a shower head filter are all it takes to eliminate most of the chlorine and other chemical exposure from tap water.

6. Maximize Your Immunity

Maximizing your immunity means using all the tools in the Living Well toolbox. Thinking Well, Eating Well, Moving Well, Sleeping Well, and Hosting Well will allow your body's natural detoxification systems to work at their best. Avoiding anti-microbial chemicals and keeping up on vaccines will help keep your immune system primed to take on the infectious threats that are part of daily life, while getting enough fiber and the good nutrition will help tap your native biological processes designed to cleanse your system every single day.

Living Well: A New Way of Life

Living Well means a whole new way of life. So let's sit back and take a look at a vibrant and successful day when it all comes together, shall we?

Imagine it's six in the morning and you've stirred a minute or two before the alarm because after the first few weeks on the program your body naturally acclimated to getting up at the same time seven days a week. You spend a few minutes in relaxed, grateful meditation and then hop out of bed, not the least bit tired—after all, you went to bed eight hours ago and quickly fell into a deep, refreshing sleep. The alarm clock is just a back-up these days—you turn it off and throw on some exercise clothes.

A few minutes later, you're outside, enjoying the early sunlight on a brisk, half-hour walk around the neighborhood. If you weren't already feeling charged up for the day, the light from the morning sun is doing the job.

Back home, after removing your shoes and leaving them at the door, you have some coffee and go over your task lists for the day. You put a big asterisk by the most important task on your list, maybe another by something you know you dread doing. Better tackle those first thing when you get to the office.

After a chlorine-free shower and a change of clothes, you have breakfast—following about twelve hours of fasting since dinner last night, you have a healthy appetite. This morning you're having organic oatmeal with organic walnuts, raspberries, and almond milk. It's one of several healthy breakfasts you enjoy in rotation to maximize the variety of foods you eat. Eating it with your family gives everyone a chance to connect and discuss their coming day. Sure, you're all busy, but even just a few minutes of chatting together and enjoying a healthy meal helps synch you up and remember what life's all about.

At work, while others are getting mired in email and social media, you're hammering down that most important task on your list. You finish more quickly than you expected thanks to a great night's sleep and few distractions. Your stand-up desk also helps keep you from getting into a mid-morning slump. You press on through that task you were dreading and when it's done, suddenly the rest of your day looks easier. You take your scheduled time to address your emails and texts and clear out your inbox just in time for lunch.

You join some co-workers and suggest a restaurant that's about a ten-minute walk away. The fresh air and sunlight recharge you and everyone really enjoys the movement and the chance to talk. You feel more like a team and you even learn a few things about your next big project that you would have never heard in a conference room meeting. For lunch you enjoy a big spinach salad with chicken, almonds, orange slices, and feta cheese crumbles, along with rustic whole wheat bread dipped in olive oil and balsamic vinegar, all of it organically sourced. Delicious! You quickly note what you ate in your food journal just to help you stay mindful of your weight loss goals.

With your most challenging tasks out of the way and your task list to guide you, the rest of the workday is a breeze. You clear out your responsibilities and even make a little headway on a pet project before heading for the community pool for a 30-minute swim. Then it's a delicious snack of yogurt and blueberries to recharge and feed your microbes.

On the way home, you stop at the grocery store and stock up on a few things you need. You spend most of your time in the organic produce aisle, choosing cabbage, broccoli, sweet potatoes, bell peppers, strawberries, apples, persimmons, and other mouth-watering produce for your family's upcoming meals. You buy some nice selections of organic meats, but also lentils and beans to pair with quinoa or brown rice as alternative proteins for a few dinners. And of course, you're almost out of extra virgin olive oil. You go through that stuff like crazy! At checkout, you notice that even with the extra cost of the organic foods, by eating so many more vegetables than meat and by substituting with legumes and other proteins, your grocery bill is about the same as it used to be before you started the Living Well Diet.

At home, you leave your shoes at the door and wash the outside germs and chemicals off your hands. You have an early dinner with your family and catch up on everyone's day and plans. With the TV off and everyone's digital devices powered down, you have a chance to really connect, laugh, and enjoy each other's company around the table with a great meal. Add a glass or two of good wine and some dark chocolate for dessert, and you are having a great time. You finish dinner at eight o'clock, stuffed from the meal of salmon with wild rice, squash, and beets. You won't be hungry again until morning.

Now, you lower the lights so everyone can start getting ready for sleep. For an hour the whole family plays a trivia game together. After the kids go to bed, you turn off more lights and read a book in your favorite chair under a low reading light. Before ten o'clock rolls around, you're already getting sleepy. You get ready for bed, then take a few minutes to write down a couple of your big accomplishments of the day—almost an hour of walking plus 30 minutes of swimming. You also made some other progress on things that are harder to quantify but still important to you and reaching your goals. Your daughter has been asking for a family game night for a while and you were glad no one had meetings or too much homework tonight. You also remember the progress you made on that pet project for work.

You get in bed at ten feeling like you accomplished a lot today in all areas of your life: family, career, fitness, and diet. You turn off the light, feeling happy. You're no longer just making it through the day. You are working toward the goals you've chosen as important to you. You're healthy, fit and well rested so you have the energy to go after what you want and it feels great to make progress every day.

Now you're not just living, you're *Living Well*.

Acknowledgements

"The truth is like a lion. You don't have do defend it. Let it loose, it will defend itself."

— St. Augustine

The truth is I started this book right after leaving GNC in 2002 and finished it in 2016. It turns out that the extra few years were very good for the final product. Some of the recommendations in the early drafts (like stand-up desks) were ten years before their time and are now popular in the mainstream. But many others have had new and strong scientific validation fairly recently, adding weight to some of the recommendations and causing revisions to some others.

Over that long and non-continuous time period of working on the ideas and the Pillars of the art and science of Living Well, I have had a lot of help in researching, improving, refining, and documenting the ideas that made this final form. My intelligent and insightful brother Douglas is the best collaborator / researcher / writer / producer anyone could hope for on this type of project. Lisa Cagle and the team at Specialty Nutrition Group have suffered through endless conversations about some pretty arcane health topics and are still smiling. Dr. Susan Trimbo provides me with regular insights into what is real and what is not in the complex field of scientific nutrition. Tom Foerstel and his creative and insightful team make everything we do look fantastic. Lisa Pineiro and Roberta Modena have been excellent editors, challenging me to make the advice relevant to busy people who are not necessarily nutrition experts.

Finally, ever since we met on her very first day of college, my brilliant and energetic wife Laura's commitment to living a purposeful life has served as a constant source of inspiration.

Resource Guide

I have prepared a comprehensive guide to tools and information resources for living your best life. This resource guide is kept updated with new insights and information at www.Living-Well.com.

References

I've cited the following studies and articles within the text. These references are great resources to learn more about particular areas of interest. I've tried to give as much information as possible in the citations so that you can easily find the studies for yourself. The vast majority of these articles and studies are at your fingertips just by entering this information into Google, Bing or another web search engine. I find this fascinating reading and I hope that you will as well.

Footnotes

[1]   Unsaturated fats are generally liquid at room temperature as opposed to saturated fats, which are generally solid.

[2]   Interestingly, about 75% of Americans have this mutation. Worldwide, however, 75% of the population do not have it because of large numbers of people from areas like Asia, where the mutation did not arise or gain prominence.

[3]   The Paleo Diet has many different permutations, permitting and omitting a variety of foods while remaining in a "Paleo Diet" core.

[4]   These results are more modest than the 2013 *New England Journal of Medicine* findings, probably reflecting the broader population studied. The diet likely had a more pronounced protective effect in the *NEJM* study because it was tested on an older population with numerous existing risk factors.

[5]   The French Paradox is that French people have a much lower incidence of coronary heart disease and tend to be thinner than one would expect, given their high intake of saturated fat. Possible explanations include protective antioxidants from wine in the diet, high intake of fruits and vegetables, probiotics from fermented cheese, and slower, more social eating.

[6]   This is only productive time as measured in a typical full time workday. Across the entire day, this person gets seven hours of sleep he has 17 hours of wakeful, productive time in his day. If the same person starts to get eight hours, he then has 16 hours of wakeful, productive time. However, in each of those 16 hours, the well-rested person is able to accomplish 25% more for the equivalent of 20 hours of productivity compared to 17 hours of productivity at the seven-hour-per-night level so the productivity gain is even greater across the entire day.

[7]   Even though there are more of these cells in *number* because our human cells are so much larger, they take up vastly more space.

[8]   Bacteria possess the ability to pass genes between themselves (even different genera and species) and mutate asexually.

[9]   The interaction of the gut flora and our immune systems are a bit too complex for this book. I can't recommend a good "short version" of the story of how our bodies and these microbes co-evolved and benefit each other. However, it is *fascinating* stuff, and I highly recommend that you read about this further, if it interests you.

[10] Often, supermarket pickles, sauerkraut, and kimchi are sterilized for commercial sale. Specialty markets and natural food stores are more likely sources for unsterilized foods. These foods don't really need sterilization, because the probiotics preserve them. And you can always make your own.

[11] Although Dr. Semmelweis's theories greatly reduced the outbreak of Childbed Fever (puerpernal fever) at his clinic, they were not widely accepted. He was ultimately committed to an insane asylum, where he was quickly killed by the guards—all around the same time that Louis Pasteur was conducting experiments that would eventually help lead to the general acceptance of "germ theory" as the primary cause of infectious diseases.

[12] I have a hard time using the term "conventionally grown" without quotation marks. This is because organic farming is much more in tune with practices of farming and land stewardship that were the convention for centuries until about 100 years ago when chemical fertilizers and sprays were introduced. They have now become the norm for agribusiness and are widely called "conventional farming" but I personally think of organic farming as more conventional and the other type as "chemical farming."

Endnotes

1. Living Well: My Story

[1] Dufty, William. *Sugar Blues*. Cancer Book House. 1975. (Current edition published by Warner Books, NY)

2. Living Well: The Program

[2] Pruitt KD, Tatusova T, Klimke W, Maglott DR. "NCBI Reference Sequences: current status, policy and new initiatives." *Nucleic Acids Res*. 2009. pp. D32–D36.

3. Grone BP, Chang D, Bourgin P, Cao V, Fernald RD, Heller HC, Ruby NF. "Acute light exposure suppresses circadian rhythms in clock gene expression." *J Biol Rhythms*. 2011 Feb26(1):78-81.

Pillar One: Thinking Well

4. Kong A, Beresford SA, Alfano CM, Foster-Schubert KE, Neuhouser ML, Johnson DB, Duggan C, Wang CY, Xiao L, Jeffery RW, Bain CE, McTiernan A. "Self-monitoring and eating-related behaviors are associated with 12-month weight loss in postmenopausal overweight-to-obese women." *J Acad Nutr Diet*. 2012 Sep112(9):1428-35.

5. Jack F. Hollis, Christina M. Gullion, Victor J. Stevens, Phillip J. Brantley, Lawrence J. Appel, Jamy D. Ard, Catherine M. Champagne, Arlene Dalcin, Thomas P. Erlinger, Kristine Funk, Daniel Laferriere, Pao-Hwa Lin, Catherine M. Loria, Carmen Samuel-Hodge, William M. Vollmer, Laura P. Svetkey and Weight Loss Maintenance Trial Research Group. "Weight Loss During the Intensive Intervention Phase of the Weight-Loss Maintenance Trial." *American Journal of*

Preventive Medicine Volume 35, Issue 2, Pages 118-126 (August 2008)

6. Larose JG, Fava JL, Steeves EA, Hecht J, Wing RR, Raynor HA. "Daily Self-Weighing Within a Lifestyle Intervention: Impact on Disordered Eating Symptoms." Health Psychol. 2013 Nov 18. [Epub ahead of print].

7. Steinberg DM, Tate DF, Bennett GG, Ennett S, Samuel-Hodge C, Ward DS. "The efficacy of a daily self-weighing weight loss intervention using smart scales and e-mail." Obesity (Silver Spring). 2013 Sep;21(9):1789-97.

8. Harkin B, Webb TL, Chang BPI, Prestwich A, Conner M, Kellar I, Benn Y, Sheeran P. "Does Monitoring Goal Progress Promote Goal Attainment? A Meta-Analysis of the Experimental Evidence." Psychological Bulletin, 2015.

9. Rubinstein, Joshua S.; Meyer, David E.; Evans, Jeffrey E. (2001). "Executive Control of Cognitive Processes in Task Switching." Journal of Experimental Psychology: Human Perception and Performance, 27(4), 763-797.

10. Park, Bum Jin; Yuko Tsunetsugu; Tamami Kasetani; Takahide Kagawa; Yoshifumi Miyazaki (2 May 2010). "The physiological effects of Shinrin-yoku (taking in the forest atmosphere or forest bathing): evidence from field experiments in 24 forests across Japan". Environmental Health and Preventive Medicine 15 (1): 18–26.

11. Lauran Donnelly, "Facebook and Twitter feed anxiety, study finds." The Telegraph July 8, 2012. http://www.telegraph.co.uk/technology/9383609/Facebook-and-Twitter-feed-anxiety-study-finds.html

12. Ricard, Matthieu. "The Habits of Happiness." TED.com. http://www.ted.com/talks/matthieu_ricard_on_the_habits_of_happiness.

Pillar Two: Eating Well

13. "2012 Food & Health Survey: Consumer attitudes toward food safety, nutrition & health" International Food Information Council Foundation, May 2012.

14. "The U.S. Weight Loss & Diet Control Market", Market Data Enterprises Inc. published in May 2011.

15. Last, Allen R.; Wilson, Stephen A. (2006). "Low-Carbohydrate Diets". American Family Physician 73 (11): 1942–8.

16. 2011 Agriculture Fact Book US Dept of Agriculture, 2011.

17. "State-specific trends in Fruit and Vegetable Consumption among Adults - United States, 2000-2009" Morbitity and Mortality Weekly Report, US Centers for Disease Control and Prevention, Sept. 10, 2010.

18. Pereira MA, O'Reilly E, Augustsson K, et al. Dietary fiber and risk of coronary heart disease: a pooled analysis of cohort studies. Arch Intern Med. 2004;164:370-6.

19. Rimm EB, Ascherio A, Giovannucci E, Spiegelman D, Stampfer MJ, Willett WC. Vegetable, fruit, and cereal fiber intake and risk of coronary heart disease among men. JAMA. 1996;275:447-51.

20. Institute of Medicine. "Dietary, Functional, and Total Fiber. Dietary Reference Intakes for Energy, Carbohydrate, Fiber, Fat, Fatty Acids, Cholesterol, Protein,

and Amino Acids." Washington, D. C.: National Academies Press; 2002:265-334. (National Academies Press).

21. Fryar CD, Ervin RB. "Caloric intake from fast food among adults: United States, 2007-2010." *NCHS data brief, no 114*. Hyattsville, MD: National Center for Health Statistics. 2013.

22. Schlosser, Eric, *Fast Food Nation*, Houton Mifflin 2001.

23. Johnson, Richard. "Michael Pollan: Why the family meal is crucial to civilization." *The Guardian* May 24, 2013.

24. National Research Council. *U.S. Health in International Perspective: Shorter Lives, Poorer Health*. Washington, DC: The National Academies Press, 2013.

25. National Research Council. *U.S. Health in International Perspective: Shorter Lives, Poorer Health*. Washington, DC: The National Academies Press, 2013.

26. National Health Examination Survey: 1960-1962; National Health and Nutrition Examination Survey: 1971-1974, 1979-1980, 1988-1994, 1999-2002, and 2007-2010; Data derived from Health, United States, 2011 (National Center for Health Statistics).

27. Last, Allen R.; Wilson, Stephen A. (2006). "Low-Carbohydrate Diets". American Family Physician 73 (11): 1942–8. PMID 16770923.

28. Skeaff CM, Miller J (2009). "Dietary Fat and Coronary Heart Disease: Summary of Evidence from Prospective Cohort and Randomised Controlled Trials" *Annals of Nutrition and Metabolism* 2009. 55:173–201.

29. Ascherio A, Katan MB, Zock PL, Stampfer MJ, Willett WC. "Trans fatty acids and coronary heart disease." *New England Journal of Medicine*. 1999 Jun 24; 340(25):1994-8.

30. "Guidance for Industry: Trans Fatty Acids in Nutrition Labeling, Nutrient Content Claims, Health Claims; Small Entity Compliance Guide." U.S. Food and Drug Administration. August 2003. http://www.fda.gov/Food/GuidanceRegulation/GuidanceDocumentsRegulatory Information/LabelingNutrition/ucm053479.htm

31. Siri-Tarino PW, Sun Q et al. (2010). "Meta-analysis of prospective cohort studies evaluating the association of saturated fat with cardiovascular disease." *American Journal of Clinical Nutrition*. January 13, 2010;

32. Cynthia A Daley, Amber Abbott, Patrick S Doyle, Glenn A Nader, and Stephanie Larson. "A review of fatty acid profiles and antioxidant content in grass-fed and grain-fed beef." *Nutr J.* 2010; 9: 10. Published online 2010 March 10.

33. Micha R, Wallace SK, Mozaffarian D. "Red and processed meat consumption and risk of incident coronary heart disease, stroke, and diabetes mellitus: a systematic review and meta-analysis." *Circulation*. 2010 Jun 1;121(21):2271-83.

34. Bouvard, Véronique et al. "Carcinogenicity of consumption of red and processed meat." *The Lancet Oncology* , Volume 16 , Issue 16 , 1599 - 1600

35. *USDA Agricultural Factbook 2001-2002*, United States Dept. of Agriculture.

36. Philpott, Tom. "We're Earting Less Meat—But Using More Antibiotics on Farms

Than Ever." *Mother Jones*. December 11, 2015. http://www.motherjones.com/tom-philpott/2015/12/meat-industry-still-cant-get-enough-antibiotics

37. White, David G. et al. "The Isolation of Antibiotic-Resistant Salmonella from Retail Ground Meats." *New England Journal of Medicine* 2001; 345:1147-1154October 18, 2001

38. Hsueh, P-R, et al. "Ciprofloxacin-resistant Salmonella enterica Typhimurium and Choleraesuis from Pigs to Humans, Taiwan" *Emerging Infectious Disease*. 2004 January; 10(1): 60–68.

39. Tavernise, Sabrina. "Antibiotics in Animals Tied to Risk of Human Infection." *The New York Times*. Jan 27, 2014.

40. "State-Specific Trends in Fruit and Vegetable Consumption Among Adults United States, 2000-2009." United States Center for Disease Control http://www.healthaliciousness.com/blog/US-fruit-vegetable-consumption-trends.php.

41. Jensen, Tom (26 February 2013). "Food issues polarizing America". *Public Policy Polling*. Retrieved 28 February 2013.

42. "Vegetarianism in America" *Vegetarian Times* 2008.

43. In Hwa Choi, Jeong Sook Noh, Ji-Sook Han, Hyun Ju Kim, Eung-Soo Han, and Yeong Ok Song. "Kimchi, a Fermented Vegetable, Improves Serum Lipid Profiles in Healthy Young Adults: Randomized Clinical Trial." *Journal of Medicinal Food*. March 2013, 16(3): 223-229.

44. Voegtlin, Walter L. *The Stone Age Diet: Based on In-depth Studies of Human Ecology and the Diet of Man*. Vantage Press, 1975

45. Cordain, Loren. *The Paleo Diet: Lose Weight and Get Healthy by Eating the Foods You Were Designed to Eat*. John Wiley & Sons, 2002

46. Lindeberg, S; & Lundh, B (March 1993). "Apparent absence of stroke and ischemic heart disease in a traditional Melanesian island: a clinical study in Kitava". *Journal of Internal Medicine* 233 (3): 269–75.

47. CJ, Mulcare CA, Itan, Y, Thomas MG, Swallow DM. "Lactose digestion and the evolutionary genetics of lactase persistence." *Hum Genet*. 2009 Jan;124(6):579-91. Ingram.

48. Enattah NE, et al. "Independent introduction of two lactase-persistence alleles into human populations reflects different history of adaptation to milk culture." *Am J Hum Genet*. 2008 Jan;82(1):57-72.

49. Dolores R. Piperno, Ehud Weiss, Irene Holst & Dani Nadel. "Processing of wild cereal grains in the Upper Palaeolithic revealed by starch grain analysis." *Nature* 430, 670-673(5 August 2004)

50. Keys A, et al. *Seven Countries. A multivariate analysis of death and coronary heart disease*. Cambridge, MA; Harvard University Press, 1980

51. Estruch, Ramón et al (February 25, 2013). "Primary Prevention of Cardiovascular Disease with a Mediterranean Diet." New England Journal of Medicine.

52. Martínez-González MA, de la Fuente-Arrillaga C, Nunez-Cordoba JM, et al. (June 2008). "Adherence to Mediterranean diet and risk of developing diabetes: prospective cohort study". *BMJ* 336 (7657): 1348–51.

53. Sofi F, Cesari F, Abbate R, Gensini GF, Casini A (2008). "Adherence to Mediterranean diet and health status: meta-analysis." *BMJ* (Clinical research ed.) 337 (sep11 2): a1344.

54. Pontin, Jason. "An Age-Defying Quest (Red Wine Included)." *The New York Times*. July 9, 2007. http://www.nytimes.com/2007/07/08/business/yourmoney/08stream.html

55. Ghanim H, Sia CL, Abuaysheh S, Korzeniewski K, Patnaik P, Marumganti A, Chaudhuri A, Dandona P. "An antiinflammatory and reactive oxygen species suppressive effects of an extract of Polygonum cuspidatum containing resveratrol." *Journal of Clinical Endocrinology and Metabolism.* 2010 Sep;95(9):E1-8.

56. Petyaev, I.M. "Carotenoid particles and uses thereof," August 2012, WO 2012/104576. International application number PCT/GD2012/00075.

57. Yuriy K. Bashmakov, Samir H. Assaad-Khalil, Myriam Abou Seif, Ruzan Udumyan, Magdy Megallaa, Kamel H. Rohoma, Mohamed Zeitoun, and Ivan M. Petyaev Clinical Study: "Resveratrol Promotes Foot Ulcer Size Reduction in Type 2 Diabetes Patients." *ISRN Endocrinology* Volume 2014 (2014), Article ID 816307. Available at: http://dx.doi.org/10.1155/2014/816307

58. Giovannucci E, Ascherio A, Rimm EB, Stampfer MJ, Colditz GA, Willett WC. "Intake of carotenoids and retinol in relation to risk of prostate cancer." *Journal of the National Cancer Institue.* 1995 Dec 6;87(23):1767-76.

59. Rissanen TH, Voutilainen S, Nyyssönen K, Salonen R, Kaplan GA, Salonen JT. "Serum lycopene concentrations and carotid atherosclerosis: the Kuopio Ischaemic Heart Disease Risk Factor Study." *American Journal of Clinical Nutrition.* 2003 Jan;77(1):133-8.

60. Estruch R., Ros E., Salas-Salvadó J., Covas M.I., Corella D., Arós F., Gómez-Gracia E., Ruiz-Gutiérrez V., Fiol M., Lapetra J., Lamuela-Raventos R.M., Serra-Majem L., Pintó X., Basora J., Muñoz M.A., Sorlí J.V., Martínez J.A., Martínez-González M.A. "Primary prevention of cardiovascular disease with a Mediterranean diet." *New England Journal of Medicine.* 2013;368:1279–1290.

61. Bitler CM, Viale TM, Damaj B, Crea R. "Hydrolyzed olive vegetation water in mice has anti-inflammatory activity." *Journal of Nutrition* 2005. 135: 1475–1479.

62. Schaffer S, Müller WE, Eckert GP. "Cytoprotective effects of olive mill wastewater extract and its main constituent hydroxytyrosol in PC12 cells." *Pharmacological Research.* 2010 Oct;62(4):322-7.

63. Estruch R., Ros E., Salas-Salvadó J., Covas M.I., Corella D., Arós F., Gómez-Gracia E., Ruiz-Gutiérrez V., Fiol M., Lapetra J., Lamuela-Raventos R.M., Serra-Majem L., Pintó X., Basora J., Muñoz M.A., Sorlí J.V., Martínez J.A., Martínez-González M.A. "Primary prevention of cardiovascular disease with a Mediterranean diet." *New England Journal of Medicine.* 2013;368:1279–1290.

64. Gadsby, Patricia (October 1, 2004). "The Inuit Paradox". *Discover Magazine*. pp. 1–4. Retrieved 24 December 2009.

65. DiMeglio DP, Mattes RD. "Liquid versus solid carbohydrate: effects on food intake and body weight." *Int J Obes Relat Metab Disord*. 2000 Jun;24(6):794-800. Available at: http://www.ncbi.nlm.nih.gov/pubmed/10878689

66. Babey SH, Jones M, Yu H, Goldstein H. "New research shows direct link between soda and obesity." *UCLA Health Policy Research* (website). 2009. Available at: http://www.healthpolicy.ucla.edu/pubs/Publication.aspx?pubID =375.

67. Natalie Zmuda. "Bottom's Up! A Look at America's Drinking Habits" *Advertising Age*, June 27, 2011,

68. Sara N. Bleich, Julia A. Wolfson, Seanna Vine, and Y. Claire Wang. "Diet-Beverage Consumption and Caloric Intake Among US Adults, Overall and by Body Weight." *American Journal of Public Health*. (2014).

69. S.E. Swithers, T.L. Davidson. "A Role for Sweet Taste: Calorie Predictive Relations in Energy Regulation by Rats." *Behavioral Neuroscience*. February 2008, Volume 122, Number 1.

70. Shapiro et al. "Fructose-Induced Leptin Resistance Exacerbates Weight Gain in Response to Subsequent High Fat Feeding." *AJP Regulatory Integrative and Comparative Physiology*, October, 2008.

71. Quanhe Yang et al. "Added Sugar Intake and Cardiovascular Diseases Mortality Among US Adults." *JAMA Intern Med*. Published online February 03, 2014.

72. Matias I, Bisogno T, Di Marzo V. "Endogenous cannabinoids in the brain and peripheral tissues: regulation of their levels and control of food intake." *International Journal of Obesity* (London). 2006 Apr;30 Suppl 1:S7-S12.

73. Guallar-Castillion P, et al. "Consumption of fried foods and risk of coronary heart disease: Spanish cohort of the European Prospective Investigation into Cancer and Nutrition study." *BMJ*. 2012 Jan 23;344:e363.

74. Estruch, Ramón et al "Primary Prevention of Cardiovascular Disease with a Mediterranean Diet". *New England Journal of Medicine*. (February 25, 2013).

75. Holahan, Charles J et al. "Late⬚Life Alcohol Consumption and 20⬚Year Mortality." *Alcoholism: Clinical and Experimental Research* 2010 Vol: 34(11):1961-1971.

76. Corrao G, Rubbiati L, Bagnardi V, Zambon A, Poikolainen K. "Alcohol and coronary heart disease: a meta-analysis." *Addiction.* 2000 Oct;95(10):1505-23.

77. Rimm EB, Klatsky A, Grobbee D, Stampfer MJ. (1996). "Review of moderate alcohol consumption and reduced risk of coronary heart disease: Is the effect due to beer, wine or spirits?" *British Medical Journal*, 312(7033):731-736.

78. Hoffmeister H, Schelp F-P, Mensink GBM, Dietz E, Bohning D. (1999). "The relationship between alcohol consumption, health indicators and mortality in the German population." *International Journal of Epidemiology*, 28(6):1066-1072.

79. McElduff P, Dobson AJ (1997). "How much alcohol and how often? Population based case control study of alcohol consumption and risk of a major coronary event." *British Medical Journal*, 314:1159-1164.

80. Jürgen Rehm, Ph.D., Gerhard Gmel, Ph.D., Christopher T. Sempos, Ph.D., and Maurizio Trevisan, M.D., M.S. "Alcohol–Related Morbidity and Mortality." *Alcohol Research & Health*. 2003 Dec;27(1);39-51.

81. Knight EL, Stampfer MJ, Hankinson SE, Spiegelman D, Curhan GC. "The impact of protein intake on renal function decline in women with normal renal function or mild renal insufficiency."*Annals of Internal Medicine*. 2003 Mar 18; 138(6):460-7.

82. Hanna Fernemark , Christine Jaredsson , Bekim Bunjaku, Ulf Rosenqvist, Fredrik H. Nystrom, Hans Guldbrand. "A Randomized Cross-Over Trial of the Postprandial Effects of Three Different Diets in Patients with Type 2 Diabetes." *PLOS One*. November 27, 2013

83. Klempel MC, Kroeger CM, Bhutani S, Trepanowski JF, Varady KA. "Intermittent fasting combined with calorie restriction is effective for weight loss and cardio-protection in obese women." *Nutr J*. 2012 Nov 21;11:98.

84. Heilbronn LK, Civitarese AE, Bogacka I, Smith SR, Hulver M, Ravussin E. "Glucose tolerance and skeletal muscle gene expression in response to alternate day fasting." *Obes Res*. 2005 Mar;13(3):574-81.

85. Sushil Kumar, Gurcharan Kaur. "Intermittent Fasting Dietary Restriction Regimen Negatively Influences Reproduction in Young Rats: A Study of Hypothalamo-Hypophysial-Gonadal Axis." *PLOS One*. January 29, 2013

86. Liu J, Hwang WT, Dickerman B, Compher C. "Regular breakfast consumption is associated with increased IQ in kindergarten children." *Early Hum Dev*. 2013 Apr;89(4):257-62.

Pillar Three: Moving Well

87. "Neural response to pictures of food after exercise in normal-weight and obese women." *Med Sci Sports Exerc*. 2012 Oct;44(10):1864-70.

88. Van Proeyen K, Szlufcik K, Nielens H, et al. "Training in the fasted state improves glucose tolerance during fat-rich diet."*Journal of Physiology*. 2010 Nov 1;588(Pt 21):4289-302.

89. Farah, NM; Gill, JM. "Effects of exercise before or after meal ingestion on fat balance and postprandial metabolism in overweight men."*Br J Nutr*. 2013 Jun 28;109(12):2297-307.

90. Van Proeyen K, Szlufcik K, Nielens H, et al. "Training in the fasted state improves glucose tolerance during fat-rich diet."*Journal of Physiology*. 2010 Nov 1;588(Pt 21):4289-302.

91. (*Medicine & Science in Sports & Exercise*, August 2010).

92. Cribb PJ, Hayes A. "Effects of supplement timing and resistance exercise on skeletal muscle hypertrophy." *Med Sci Sports Exerc*. 2006 Nov;38(11):1918-25.

93. Katie Adolphus, Clare L. Lawton, Louise Dye. "The effects of breakfast on behavior and academic performance in children and adolescents." *Front Hum Neurosci*. 2013; 7: 425.

94. Farah NMF, et al. "Effects of exercise before or after meal ingestion on fat balance and postprandial metabolism in overweight men." *British Journal of Nutrition*. Published online: 26 October 2012

95. Hill, DW. "Temporal specificity in adaptations to high-intensity exercise training." *Med Sci Sports Exerc*. 1998 Mar;30(3):450-5.

96. Nam J et al. "Transcriptome-wide gene regulation by gentle treadmill walking during the progression of monoiodoacetate-induced arthritis." *Arthritis & Rheumatism*. Volume 63, Issue 6, pages 1613–1625, June 2011

97. Comuzzie AG, Allison DB. "The Search for Human Obesity Genes." *Science* 29 Vol. 280, Issue 5368, pp. 1374-1377. May 1998

98. American Heart Association's 2012 meeting on Epidemiology and Prevention/Nutrition, Physical Activity and Metabolism

99. Wallace. *Journal of Hypertension*, Sept. 2006.

100. Möhlenkamp et al, 2008 European Heart Journal & Breuckmann et al., 2009 Radiology

101. James H. O'Keefe. "Potential Adverse Cardiovascular Effects From Excessive Endurance Exercise." *Mayo Clin Proc*. 2012 June; 87(6): 587–595.

102. "Diverse patterns of myocardial fibrosis in lifelong, veteran endurance athletes." *J Appl Physiol*. 2011 June; 110(6): 1622–1626

103. Lee DC, Pate RR, Lavie CJ, et al. "Running and all-cause mortality risk—is more better?" *American College of Sports Medicine* 2012 Annual Meeting; June 2, 2012; San Francisco, CA. Presentation 3471.

104. Lee DC, Pate RR, Lavie CJ, et al. "Running and all-cause mortality risk—is more better?" *American College of Sports Medicine* 2012 Annual Meeting; June 2, 2012; San Francisco, CA. Presentation 3471.

105. *Arteriosclerosis, Thrombosis, and Vascular Biology* in April 2013,

106. *Medicine & Science in Sports & Exercise*, February 2013

107. *British Journal of Sports Medicine*, March 2013.

108. Zipfel, B.; L.R. Berger. "Shod versus unshod: The emergence of forefoot pathology in modern humans?" *The Foot*.

109. Brown D, Chevalier G, Hill M. "Pilot study on the effect of grounding on delayed-onset muscle soreness." *J Altern Complement Med*. 2010 Mar; 16(3):265-73.

110. Google Dictionary definition. https://www.google.com/#q=definition:+sedentary

111. Biswas A, Oh PI, Faulkner GE, Bajaj R.R., Silver MA, Mitchell MS, and Alter DA. "Sedentary Time and Its Association With Risk for Disease Incidence, Mortality, and Hospitalization in Adults: A Systematic Review and Meta-analysis". *Annals of Internal Medicine*, 2015

112. Bey L, Hamilton MT. "Suppression of skeletal muscle lipoprotein lipase activity during physical inactivity: a molecular reason to maintain daily low-intensity activity." *J Physiol* 2003, 551:673-682

113. Tatiana Y. Warren, Vaughn Barry, Steven P. Hooker, Xuemei Sui, Timothy S. Church, Steven N. Blair. "Sedentary Behaviors Increase Risk of Cardiovascular Disease Mortality in Men." *Med Sci Sports Exerc.* 2010 May; 42(5): 879-885.

114. Wimot EG, Edwardson CL, Achana FA, et al. "Sedentary time in adults and the association with diabetes, cardiovascular disease and death: Systematic review and meta-analysis." *Diabetologia* 2012; 55:2895-2905.

115. Craft et al. "Evidence that women meeting physical activity guidelines do not sit less: An observational inclinometry study." *International Journal of Behavioral Nutrition and Physical Activity* 2012, 9:122 http://www.ijbnpa.org/content/9/1/122

116. Katzmarzyk, Dr. Peter and Lee, I-Min. "Sedentary behaviour and life expectancy in the USA: a cause-deleted life table analysis." *BMJ Open* 2012;2:e000828

117. Ekblom-Bak E, Ekblom B, Vikström M, et al. "The importance of non-exercise physical activity for cardiovascular health and longevity." [Journal Article] *Br J Sports Med* 2014 Feb; 48(3):233-8.

118. Beers, E. A. et al. 2008. "Increasing passive energy expenditure during clerical work." *European Journal of Applied Physiology* 103: 353-360

119. http://bjsm.bmj.com/content/46/13/927.full

120. http://www.nydailynews.com/entertainment/tv-movies/americans-spend-34-hours-week-watching-tv-nielsen-numbers-article-1.1162285

121. USMS Swimmer, Latina, Raena Alexis. "Fountain of Youth: Researcher explores relationship between swimming and aging." http://www.usms swimmer.com/200607/fountainofyouth.pdf

122. Stager/Tanner. (2005). *Handbook on Sports Medicine and Science: Swimming.* London: Blackwell Scientific.

123. Tanaka H and colleagues. Swimming training lowers the resting blood pressure in individuals with hypertension. *Journal of Hypertension* 1997;15:651-57.

124. Westby, MD. "A health professional's guide to exercise prescription for people with arthritis: a review of aerobic fitness activities." *Arthritis Care and Res.* 2001. 45(6):501-11.

125. Bartels EM, Lund H, Hagen KB, Dagfinrud H, Christensen R, Danneskiold-Samsøe B. 2007. "Aquatic exercise for the treatment of knee and hip osteoarthritis." *Cochrane Database of Systematic Reviews.* 4:1-9.

126. Hall J, Skevington SM, Maddison PJ, and Chapman K. 1996. "A randomized and controlled trial of hydrotherapy in rheumatoid arthritis." *Arthritis Care Res.* 9(3):206-15.

127. Hall J, Skevington SM, Maddison PJ, Chapman K. "A randomized and controlled trial of hydrotherapy in rheumatoid arthritis." *Arthritis Care and Research.* 1996 Jun;9(3):206-15.

128. Sato D, Kaneda K, Wakabayashi H, and Nomura T. 2007. "The water exercise improves health-related quality of life of frail elderly people at day service facility." *Qual Life Res*. 16:1577-85.

129. Rotstein A, Harush M, and Vaisman N. 2008. "The effect of water exercise program on bone density of postmenopausal Women." *J Sports Med Phys Fitness*. 48(3):352-9.

130. Berger BG, and Owen DR. 1992. "Mood alteration with yoga and swimming: aerobic exercise may not be necessary." *Percept Mot Skills*. 75(3 Pt 2):1331-43.

131. Pöyhönen T, Sipilä S, Keskinen KL, et al. "Effects of aquatic resistance training on neuromuscular performance in healthy women." *Medicine & Science in Sports & Exercise*. 2002. 34:2103-2109.

132. Takeshima N, Rogers ME, Watanabe E, et al. "Water-based exercise improves health-related aspects of fitness in older women." *Medicine & Science in Sports & Exercise*. 2002. 33:544-551.

133. Jonatan R Ruiz, Xuemei Sui, Felipe Lobelo, James R Morrow Jr, Allen W Jackson, Michael Sjo¨stro¨m, Steven N Blair. "Association between muscular strength and mortality in men: prospective cohort study." *BMJ* 2008;337:a439.

134. Bliss, Rosalie Marion. *Agricultural Research*. May 2005. Pg. 15

135. Hasten, D.L. et al. "Resistance Exercise Acutely Increases MHC and Mixed Muscle Protein Synthesis Rates in 78-84 and 23-32 yr olds." *American Journal of Physiology* 2000. 278:620-626.

136. Yarasheski, K.E. et al. 1999. "Resistance Exercise Training Increases Mixed Muscle Protein Synthesis Rate in Frail Women and Men - 76 yr old." *American Journal of Physiology* 277: 118-125.

137. Brenner C, Jaksch F, Dellinger R. "Dose-Dependent Elevation of the Blood NAD Metabolome by NR in Healthy Human Beings." Presentation at the 4th Federation of American Societies for Experimental Biology (FASEB) Science Research Conference on NAD+ Metabolism and Signaling, Aug 12, 2015 Timmendorfer Strand, Germany

138. Hespel, P; Eijnde, BO; Derave, W; Richter, EA. "Creatine supplementation: Exploring the role of the creatine kinase/phosphocreatine system in human muscle." *Canadian Journal of Applied Physiology* 26 Suppl: S79–102. (2001). Olsen, S.; Aagaard, P; Kadi, F; Tufekovic, G; Verney, J; Olesen, JL; Suetta, C; Kjaer, M. "Creatine supplementation augments the increase in satellite cell and myonuclei number in human skeletal muscle induced by strength training." *The Journal of Physiology* 573 (2): 525–34. (2006).

139. Van Der Merwe, Johann; Brooks, Naomi E; Myburgh, Kathryn H "Three Weeks of Creatine Monohydrate Supplementation Affects Dihydrotestosterone to Testosterone Ratio in College-Aged Rugby Players." *Clinical Journal of Sport Medicine* 19 (2009). (5): 399–404.

140. Burke, DG; Candow, DG; Chilibeck, PD; MacNeil, LG; Roy, BD; Tarnopolsky, MA; Ziegenfuss, T "Effect of creatine supplementation and resistance-exercise

training on muscle insulin-like growth factor in young adults." *International Journal of Sport Nutrition and Exercise Metabolism* 18 (4): 389–98. 2008.

141. Jagim AG, Oliver JM, Sanchez A, et al. "A buffered form of creatine does not promote greater changes in muscle content, body composition, or training adaptations than creatine monohydrate" *Journal of the International Society of Sports Nutrition.* 2012. 13;9(1)

142. Tarnopolsky M, Martin J. "Creatine monohydrate increases strength in patients with neuromuscular disease." *Neurology* 1999. 52:854–857.

143. Karlsson HK, Nilsson PA, Nilsson J, Chibalin AV, Zierath JR, Blomstrand E. "Branched-chain amino acids increase phosphorylation in human skeletal muscle after resistance exercise." *Am J Physiol Endocrinol Metab.* 2004 Jul;287(1):E1-7.

144. Jackman SR, Witard OC, Jeukendrup AE, Tipton KD. "Branched-chain amino acid ingestion can ameliorate soreness from eccentric exercise." *Med Sci Sports Exerc.* 2010 May;42(5):962-70.

145. Reidy PT, et al. "Protein blend ingestion following resistance exercise promotes human muscle protein synthesis." *J Nutr.* 2013 Apr;143(4):410-6.

Pillar Four: Sleeping Well

146. Jones, Jeffrey M. "In U.S., 40% Get Less Than Recommended Amount of Sleep" Gallup Well-Being Dec 19, 2013. http://www.gallup.com/poll/166553/less-recommended-amount-sleep.aspx .

147. Orzeł-Gryglewska J. "Consequences of sleep deprivation." *Int J Occup Med Environ Health.* 2010;23(1):95-114.

148. "Guidelines for the Care and Use of Mammals in Neuroscience and Behavioral Research. Institute for Laboratory Animal Research (ILAR), National Research Council. The National Academies Press. 2003. p. 121. ISBN 978-0-309-08903-6.

149. Daan S, Barnes BM, Strijkstra AM (1991). "Warming up for sleep? Ground squirrels sleep during arousals from hibernation". *Neurosci. Lett.* 128 (2): 265–8.

150. Nedergaard, Maiken et al. "Sleep Drives Metabolite Clearance from the Adult Brain." *Science* 18 October 2013: Vol. 342 no. 6156 pp. 373-377

151. Van Dongen HPA, Maislin G, Mullington JM, Dinges DF. "The cumulative cost of additional wakefulness: dose response effects on neurobehavioral functions and sleep physiology from chronic sleep restriction and total sleep deprivation." *Sleep* 2003;26:117–126.

152. Williamson, A M; Feyer, Anne-Marie. "Moderate sleep deprivation produces impairments in cognitive and motor performance equivalent to legally prescribed levels of alcohol intoxication." *Occup Environ Med* 2000;57:649–655.

153. Jones, Maggie. "How Little Sleep Can You Get Away With?" *The New York Times.* April 15, 2011.

154. Breslau N, Roth T, Rosenthal L, Andreski P. "Daytime sleepiness: an epidemiological study of young adults." *Am J Public Health* 1997; 87:1649–1653.

155. Van Dongen HP1, Maislin G, Mullington JM, Dinges DF. "The cumulative cost of additional wakefulness: dose-response effects on neurobehavioral functions and sleep physiology from chronic sleep restriction and total sleep deprivation." *Sleep*. 2003 Mar 15;26(2):117-26.

156. Gumustekin, K.; Seven, B.; Karabulut, N.; Aktas, O.; Gursan, N.; Aslan, S.; Keles, M.; Varoglu, E.; Dane, S. "Effects of sleep deprivation, nicotine, and selenium on wound healing in rats." *Int J Neurosci* 114 (11): 1433–42. 2004.

157. Opp, Mark R (January 2009). "Sleeping to fuel the immune system: mammalian sleep and resistance to parasites" *BMC Evolutionary Biology* (BioMed Central Ltd.) 9: 1471–2148.

158. Zager, A.; Andersen, M.L.; Ruiz, F.S.; Antunes, I.B. and Tufik, S. (2007). "Effects of acute and chronic sleep loss on immune modulation of rats." *Regulatory, Integrative and Comparative Physiology* 293: R504–R509.

159. Guidelines for the Care and Use of Mammals in Neuroscience and Behavioral Research. Institute for Laboratory Animal Research (ILAR), National Research Council. The National Academies Press. 2003. p. 121. ISBN 978-0-309-08903-6.

160. Van Cauter, E.; Leproult, R.; Plat, L. "Age-related changes in slow-wave sleep and REM sleep and relationship with growth hormone and cortisol levels in healthy men." *Journal of the American Medical Association* 284 (7): 861–868. 2000.

161. Taheri S, Lin L, Austin D, Young T, Mignot E (December 2004). "Short Sleep Duration Is Associated with Reduced Leptin, Elevated Ghrelin, and Increased Body Mass Index". *PLoS Med*. 1 (3): e62.

162. Moller-Levet CS, Archer SN, Bucca G, et al. "Effects of insufficient sleep on circadian rhythmicity and expression amplitude of the human blood transcriptome." *Proc Natl Acad Sci USA*. 2013;110:E1132–E1141.

163. Fairclough SH, Graham R. "Impairment of driving performance caused by sleep deprivation or alcohol: a comparative study." *Hum Factors* 1999; 41:118–128.

164. Williamson AM, Feyer AM. "Moderate sleep deprivation produces impairments in cognitive and motor performance equivalent to legally prescribed levels of alcohol intoxication." *Occup Environ Med* 2000;57:649–655.

165. Harrison Y, Horne J. "The impact of sleep deprivation on decision making: A review." *Journal of Experimental Psychology: Applied*. 6:236-249. 2000.

166. Fujikawa T., Tochikubo O., Kura N., & Umemura S. (2009). "Factors related to elevated 24-h blood pressure in young adults." *Clinical and Experimental Hypertension*, 31(8), 705-712.

167. Lusardi P., Mugellini A., Preti P., Zoppi A., Derosa G., Fogari R. "Effects of a restricted sleep regimen on ambulatory blood pressure monitoring in normotensive subjects." *Am J Hypertension*. 1996;9:503–5.

168. Pilcher, June J.; Huffcutt, Allen J. "Effects of sleep deprivation on performance: A meta-analysis." *Sleep: Journal of Sleep Research & Sleep Medicine*, Vol 19(4), May 1996, 318-326.

Pillar Five: Hosting Well

169. Born, J.; Rasch, J.; Gais, S. (2006). "Sleep to remember." *Neuroscientist* 12: 410.

170. Taheri S, Lin L, Austin D, Young T, Mignot E (December 2004). "Short Sleep Duration Is Associated with Reduced Leptin, Elevated Ghrelin, and Increased Body Mass Index". *PLoS Med*. 1 (3): e62.

171. Benedict C., Brooks S. J., O'Daly O. G., Almèn M. S., Morell A., Åberg K., ... & Schiöth H. B. "Acute sleep deprivation enhances the brain's response to hedonic food stimuli: an fMRI study." *Journal of Clinical Endocrinology & Metabolism*, 97(3), E443-E447. 2012.

172. James E. Gangwisch. "Inadequate Sleep as a Risk Factor for Obesity: Analyses of the NHANES I."*SLEEP*, Vol. 28, No. 10, 2005.

173. Nedeltcheva AV, Kilkus JM, Imperial J, Schoeller DA, Penev PD. "Insufficient sleep underminesdietary efforts to reduce adiposity." *Annals of Internal Medicine*. Oct. 5, 2010. 153(7) 435-441.

174. "Survey: Americans Crave Sleep More Than Sex." Better Sleep Council press release. 2002. http://bettersleep.org/press-room/press-releases/americans-crave-sleep-more-than-sex-says-better-sleep-council-survey.

175. Rosekind MR, Gregory KB, Mallis MM, Brandt SL, Seal B, Lerner D. "The cost of poor sleep: workplace productivity loss and associated costs." *J Occup Environ Med*. 2010 Jan;52(1):91-8.

176. Weber, Lauren. "Go Ahead, Hit the Snooze Button." *Wall Street Journal*, Jan 23, 2013. http://online.wsj.com/article/SB10001424127887323301104578257894191502654.html .

177. Vural EM, van Munster BC, de Rooij SE. "Optimal dosages for melatonin supplementation therapy in older adults: a systematic review of current literature." *Drugs Aging*. 2014 Jun;31(6):441-51.

178. Bettelheim, K. A.; Breadon, Alwena; Faiers, Mary C.; O'Farrell, Sheila M.; Shooter, R. A. "The origin of O serotypes of Escherichia coli in babies after normal delivery." *Journal of Hygiene* 72 (1): 67–70. 2009.

179. Grölund, Minna-Maija; Lehtonen, Olli-Pekka; Eerola, Erkki; Kero, Pentti "Fecal Microflora in Healthy Infants Born by Different Methods of Delivery: Permanent Changes in Intestinal Flora After Cesarean Delivery." *Journal of Pediatric Gastroenterology & Nutrition* 28 (1): 19–25. 1999.

180. Baker, Monya. "Pregnancy alters resident gut microbes." *Nature*. 2012.

181. Ward RE et al. "In Vitro fermentability of human milk oligosaccharides by several strains of bifidobacteria." *Mol. Nutr. Food Res*. 2007;51:1398-1405.

182. Schell MA et al. "The genome sequence of Bifidobacterium longum reflects its adaptation to the human gastrointestinal tract." *Proceedings of the National Academy of Sciences* 2002;99:22:14422-14427.

183. Saavedra, Jose M. "Use of Probiotics in Pediatrics: Rationale, Mechanisms of Action, and Practical Aspects." *Nutrition in Clinical Practice* 22(3), 351-365.

184. Saavedra, Jose M. "Use of Probiotics in Pediatrics: Rationale, Mechanisms of Action, and Practical Aspects." *Nutrition in Clinical Practice* 22(3), 351-3652.

185. Grice EA, Kong HH, Conlan S. "Topographical and Temporal Diversity of the Human Skin Microbiome." *Science*, 324: 1190 - 1192. 2009.

186. Kerr JR. (1994). "Suppression of fungal growth exhibited by Pseudomonas aeruginosa." *J Clin Microbiol*. 32(2):525-7.

187. Cogen AL, Nizet V, Gallo RL. (2008). "Skin microbiota: a source of disease or defence?" *Br J Dermatol*. 158(3):442-55.

188. Tap, Julien; Mondot, Stanislas; Levenez, Florence; Pelletier, Eric; Caron, Christophe; Furet, Jean-Pierre; Ugarte, Edgardo; Muñoz-Tamayo, Rafael; Paslier, Denis L. E.; Nalin, Renaud; Dore, Joel; Leclerc, Marion. "Towards the human intestinal microbiota phylogenetic core." *Environmental Microbiology* 11 (10): 2574–84. 2009.

189. Heheman HJ. "Transfer of carbohydrate-active enzymes from marine bacteria to Japanese gut microbiota." *Nature*. 2010 Apr 8;464(7290):908-12.

190. O'Hara, Ann M; Shanahan, Fergus "The gut flora as a forgotten organ." *EMBO Reports* 7 (7): 688–93. 2006.

191. Sears, Cynthia L. "A dynamic partnership: Celebrating our gut flora." *Anaerobe* 11 (5): 247–51. 2005.

192. Sears, Cynthia L. "A dynamic partnership: Celebrating our gut flora." *Anaerobe* 11 (5): 247–51. 2005.

193. Ripudaman S. Beniwal, et al., "A Randomized Trial of Yogurt for Prevention of Antibiotic-Associated Diarrhea." *Digestive Diseases and Sciences* 48:10:2077-2082 (October, 2003).

194. Burke, KE; Lamont, JT (August 2013). "Fecal Transplantation for Recurrent Clostridium difficile Infection in Older Adults: A Review." *Journal of the American Geriatrics Society* 61 (8): 1394–8.

195. Bakken, Johan S.; Borody, Thomas; Brandt, Lawrence J.; Brill, Joel V.; Demarco, Daniel C.; Franzos, Marc Alaric; Kelly, Colleen; Khoruts, Alexander; Louie, Thomas; Martinelli, Lawrence P.; Moore, Thomas A.; Russell, George; Surawicz, Christina. "Treating Clostridium difficile Infection With Fecal Microbiota Transplantation." *Clinical Gastroenterology and Hepatology* 9 (12): 1044–1049. 1 December 2011.

196. Ananthaswamy, Anil "Faecal transplant eases symptoms of Parkinson's." *New Scientist*. 19 January 2011.

197. Sears, Cynthia L. "A dynamic partnership: Celebrating our gut flora." Anaerobe 11 (5): 247–51. 2005.

198. Upton, Joanne R. (2004). "Microbial Degradation Products Influence Colon Cancer Risk: the Butyrate Controversy." *Journal of Nutrition* 134 (2): 479–82.

199. Cummings, J.H.; MacFarlane, G.T. "Role of intestinal bacteria in nutrient metabolism." *Clinical Nutrition* 16: 3–9. 1997.

200. Sugimura, T. "Nutrition and dietary carcinogens". *Carcinogenesis* 21 (3): 387–95. 2000.

201. Cho I, Yamanishi S, Cox L, Methé BA, Zavadil J, Li K, Gao Z, Mahana D, Raju K, Teitler I, Li H, Alekseyenko AV, Blaser MJ. "Antibiotics in early life alter the murine colonic microbiome and adiposity." *Nature*. 2012 Aug 30;488(7413):621-6.

202. Cho I, et al. "Antibiotics in early life alter the murine colonic microbiome and adiposity." *Nature*. 2012 Aug 30;488(7413):621-6.

203. Metcalf BS, Hosking J, Jeffery AN, Voss LD, Henley W, Wilkin TJ. "Fatness leads to inactivity, but inactivity does not lead to fatness: a longitudinal study in children." *Arch Dis Child*. 2011 Oct;96(10):942-7.

204. Ridaura VK, Faith JJ, Rey FE, Cheng J, Duncan AE, Kau AL, Griffin NW, Lombard V, Henrissat B, Bain JR, Muehlbauer MJ, Ilkayeva O, Semenkovich CF, Funai K, Hayashi DK, Lyle BJ, Martini MC, Ursell LK, Clemente JC, Van Treuren W, Walters WA, Knight R, Newgard CB, Heath AC, Gordon JI. "Gut microbiota from twins discordant for obesity modulate metabolism in mice." *Science*. 2013 Sep 6;341(6150):1241214.

205. Goodrich Julia K., Jillian L. Waters, Angela C. Poole, Jessica L. Sutter, Omry Koren, Ran Blekhman, Michelle Beaumont, William Van Treuren, Rob Knight, Jordana T. Bell, Timothy D. Spector, Andrew G. Clark, Ruth E. Ley. "Human Genetics Shape the Gut Microbiome." *Cell*, 2014 Nov 5;159(4):789–799.

206. Ghouri YA, Richards DM, Rahimi EF, Krill JT, Jelinek KA, DuPont AW. "Systematic review of randomized controlled trials of probiotics, prebiotics, and synbiotics in inflammatory bowel disease". *Clinical and Experimental Gastroenterology*. pp. 473 – 4879 December 2014

207. Basulto, Dominic. "Eating poop pills could make you thin. Seriously." *The Washington Post*. January 14, 2016. https://www.washingtonpost.com/news/innovations/wp/2016/01/14/eating-poop-pills-could-make-you-thin-seriously/

208. Messaoudi M, Lalonde R, Violle N et al. "Assessment of psychotropiclike properties of a probiotic formulation (Lactobacillus helveticus R0052 and Bifidobacterium longum R0175) in rats and human subjects." *Br J Nutr* 2010; 26: 1–9.

209. "Getting Dirty May Lift Your Mood". *Bristol University: Medical News Today*. 2007-04-05.

210. Jo WK, Weisel CP, Lioy PJ. "Chloroform exposure and the health risk associated with multiple uses of chlorinated tap water." *Risk Anal*. 1990 Dec;10(4):581-5.

211. Kuo HW, Chiang TF, Lo II, Lai JS, Chan CC, Wang JD. "Estimates of cancer risk from chloroform exposure during showering in Taiwan." *Sci Total Environ*. 1998 Jul 11;218(1):1-7.

212. Jane Zhang. "FDA questions use of antibacterial soaps." *The Wall Street Journal*. Tuesday, October 18, 2005.

213. Adolfsson-Erici M, Pettersson M, Parkkonen J, Sturve J. "Triclosan, a commonly used bactericide found in human milk and in the aquatic environment in Sweden". *Chemosphere* 46 (9–10): 1485–9. March 2002.

214. Veldhoen N, Skirrow RC, Osachoff H, et al. "The bactericidal agent triclosan modulates thyroid hormone-associated gene expression and disrupts postembryonic anuran development." *Aquat. Toxicol.* 80 (3): 217–27. December 2006.

215. F. Breidt, Jr. "A Genomic Study of Leuconostoc mesenteroides and the Molecular Ecology of Sauerkraut Fermentations." *Journal of Food Science* 69 (1): 30–33. 2004.

216. Kim EK, An SY, Lee MS, Kim TH, Lee HK, Hwang WS, Choe SJ, Kim TY, Han SJ, Kim HJ, Kim DJ, Lee KW. "Fermented kimchi reduces body weight and improves metabolic parameters in overweight and obese patients." *Nutr Res.* 2011 Jun;31(6):436-43.

217. Queipo-Ortuno, M., Boto-Ordonez, M., Murri, M., Gomez-Zumaquero, J., Clemente-Postigo, M., Estruch, R., Cardona Diaz, F., Andres-Lacueva, C., & Tinahones, F. "Influence of red wine polyphenols and ethanol on the gut microbiota ecology and biochemical biomarkers." *American Journal of Clinical Nutrition*, 95 (6), 1323-1334. 2012.

Pillar Six: Staying Well

218. Philippe Grandjean, Philip Landrigan. Neurobehavioural effects of developmental toxicity. *Lancet Neurology*, February 2014

219. Jjemot RI, Ehiri JE, Meremikwu MM, Critchley JA. "Hand washing for preventing diarrhoea." Cochrane Database Syst Rev. 2008;(1):CD004265.

220. Harnly ME, Bradman A, Nishioka M, McKone TE, Smith D, McLaughlin R, Kavanagh-Baird G, Castorina R, Eskenazi B. "Pesticides in dust from homes in an agricultural area." *Environ Sci Technol*. 2009;43(23):8767-74.

221. Barbara J. Mahler, Peter C. Van Metre, Judy L. Crane, Alison W. Watts, Mateo Scoggins, and E. Spencer Williams. "Coal-Tar-Based Pavement Sealcoat and PAHs: Implications for the Environment, Human Health, and Stormwater Management." *Environmental Science & Technology*. 2012. 46, 3039–3045.

222. Roberts, J.W. & Ott, W.R. (2007). "Exposure to Pollutants from House Dust." In Ott, W.R., Steinemann, A.C. & Wallace, L.A. (Eds.) *Exposure Analysis*, 319–345. New York: Taylor & Francis.

223. Frank D. Roylance. "The 'ewww!' on your shoe." *The Baltimore Sun*. May 8, 2008.

224. Robin McKie. "Onset of puberty in girls has fallen by five years since 1920." *The Guardian*. Oct. 20, 2012.

225. Sharpe RM. The 'oestrogen hypothesis'- where do we stand now? *Int J Androl*. 2003 Feb;26(1):2-15.

226. Grün F, Blumberg B. "Endocrine disrupters as obesogens." *Mol Cell Endocrinol*. 2009 May 25;304(1-2):19-29.

227. Cheng G, Wilczek B, Warner M, Gustafsson JA, Landgren BM. "Isoflavone treatment for acute menopausal symptoms." *Menopause*. 2007 May-Jun;14(3 Pt 1):468-73.

228. E Balk, M Chung, P Chew, S Ip, G Raman, B Kupelnick, A Tatsioni, Y Sun, D Devine, and J Lau. "Effects of Soy on Health Outcomes." Agency for Healthcare Research and Quality (US); 1998-2005

229. Allred CD, Allred KF, Ju YH, Virant SM, Helferich WG. "Soy diets containing varying amounts of genistein stimulate growth of estrogen-dependent (MCF-7) tumors in a dose-dependent manner." *Cancer Res*. 2001 Jul 1;61(13):5045-50.

230. N L Petrakis, S Barnes, E B King, J Lowenstein, J Wiencke, M M Lee, R Miike, M Kirk and L Coward. "Stimulatory influence of soy protein isolate on breast secretion in pre- and postmenopausal women." *Cancer Epidemiol Biomarkers Prev* October 1996 5; 785.

231. Danielle F McMichael-Phillips, Claudia Harding, Mike Morton, Stephen A Roberts, Anthony Howell, Christopher S Potten, and Nigel J Bundred. "Effects of soy-protein supplementation on epithelial proliferation in the histologically normal human breast." *Am J Clin Nutr* December 1998 vol. 68 no. 6 1431S-1435S.

232. Ingram D, Sanders K, Kolybaba M, Lopez D (October 1997). "Case-control study of phyto-oestrogens and breast cancer". *Lancet* 350 (9083): 990–994.

233. Hiroshi Masuno, Teruki Kidani, Keizo Sekiya, Kenshi Sakayama, Takahiko Shiosaka, Haruyasu Yamamoto, and Katsuhisa Honda. "Bisphenol A in combination with insulin can accelerate the conversion of 3T3-L1 fibroblasts to adipocytes." May 2002 *The Journal of Lipid Research*, 43, 676-684.

234. Lang IA, Galloway TS, Scarlett A, Henley WE, Depledge M, Wallace RB, Melzer D (2008). "Association of Urinary Bisphenol A Concentration With Medical Disorders and Laboratory Abnormalities in Adults". *JAMA* 300 (11): 1303–10.

235. Meeker, John D.; Calafat, Antonia M.; Hauser, Russ (2010). "Urinary Bisphenol a Concentrations in Relation to Serum Thyroid and Reproductive Hormone Levels in Men from an Infertility Clinic". *Environmental Science & Technology 44 (4): 1458.*

236. Li DK, Zhou Z, Miao M, He Y, Qing D, Wu T, Wang J, Weng X, Ferber J, Herrinton LJ, Zhu Q, Gao E, Yuan W (2010). "Relationship between urine bisphenol-A level and declining male sexual function". *J. Androl*. 31 (5): 500–6.

237. Sugiura-Ogasawara, M.; Ozaki, Y; Sonta, S; Makino, T; Suzumori, K (2005). "Exposure to bisphenol a is associated with recurrent miscarriage". *Human Reproduction* 20 (8): 2325–9.

238. Clayton, EM; Todd, M; Dowd, JB; Aiello, AE (2011). "The impact of bisphenol a and triclosan on immune parameters in the U.S. Population, NHANES 2003-2006". *Environmental health perspectives* 119 (3): 390–6.

239. Duan B, Hu X, Zhao H, Qin J, Luo J (April 2012). "The relationship between urinary bisphenol A levels and meningioma in Chinese adults". *Int J Clin Oncol* 18 (3): 492–7.

240. Brisken, Cathrin (2008). "Endocrine Disruptors and Breast Cancer". *CHIMIA International Journal for Chemistry* 62 (5): 406.

241. Leranth C, Hajszan T, Szigeti-Buck K, Bober J, Maclusky NJ (September 2008). "Bisphenol A prevents the synaptogenic response to estradiol in hippocampus and prefrontal cortex of ovariectomized nonhuman primates". *Proc. Natl. Acad. Sci. U.S.A.* 105 (37): 14187–91.

242. Wolstenholme JT, et al (2012) Gestational exposure to bisphenol a produces transgenerational changes in behaviors and gene expression. *Endocrinology.* 153(8):3828-38.

243. Janet Ralof. "Concerned about BPA: Check your receipts." *Science News.* October 7, 2009.

244. Desvergne B, Feige J, Casals-Casas C (2009). "PPAR-mediated activity of phthalates: A link to the obesity epidemic?". *Mol Cell Endocrinol.* 304 (1–2): 43–8.

245. Albert, O.; Jegou, B. (2013). "A critical assessment of the endocrine susceptibility of the human testis to phthalates from fetal life to adulthood". *Human Reproduction Update* 20 (2): 231.

246. Lopez-Carillo L., Hernandez-Ramirez R.U., Calafat A.M., Torres-Sanchez L., Galvan-Portillo M., Needham L.L., Ruiz-Ramos R., Cebrian M.E. (2010). "Exposure to phthalates and breast cancer risk in Northern Mexico". *Environmental Health Perspectives* 114 (4): 539–544.

247. Bornehag CG, Sundell J, Weschler CJ, Sigsgaard T, Lundgren B, Hasselgren M, Hägerhed-Engman L (October 2004). "The Association between Asthma and Allergic Symptoms in Children and Phthalates in House Dust: A Nested Case–Control Study". *Environ. Health Perspect.* 112 (14): 1393–7.

248. "Phthalates in PVC floors taken up by the body in infants". *Sciencedaily.com.* 2012-05-23.

249. Yang CZ, Yaniger SI, Jordan VC, Klein DJ, Bittner GD. "Most plastic products release estrogenic chemicals: a potential health problem that can be solved." *Environ Health Perspect.* 2011 Jul;119(7):989-96.

250. Crinnion WJ. "Organic foods contain higher levels of certain nutrients, lower levels of pesticides, and may provide health benefits for the consumer."*Altern Med Rev.* 2010 Apr;15(1):4-12.

251. John P. Reganold, Preston K. Andrews, Jennifer R. Reeve, Lynne Carpenter-Boggs, Christopher W. Schadt, J. Richard Alldredge, Carolyn F. Ross,Neal M. Davies, Jizhong Zhou. "Fruit and Soil Quality of Organic and Conventional Strawberry Agroecosystems." *PLoS One.* September 01, 2010

252. Sabrina Tavernise. "Study Finds an Increase in Arsenic Levels in Chicken". *The New York Times.* May 11, 2013.

253. Te-Ping Chen. "Threat to Rice Fuels Latest Chinese Uproar Guangzhou Finds High Cadmium Levels In New Scare Over Contaminated Food." *The Wall Street Journal.* May 21, 2013.

254. Vahter M, Berglund M, Nermell B, Akesson A. "Bioavailability of cadmium from shellfish and mixed diet in women." *Toxicol Appl Pharmacol*. 1996 Feb;136(2):332-41.

255. Needleman HL, Gatsonis CA. "Low-Level Lead Exposure and the IQ of Children: A Meta-analysis of Modern Studies."*Journal of the American Medical Association*. 1990;263(5):673-678

256. The Editors Of The Lancet (February 2010). "Retraction – Ileal-lymphoid-nodular hyperplasia, non-specific colitis, and pervasive developmental disorder in children". *The Lancet* 375 (9713): 445.

257. Godlee F, Smith J, Marcovitch H (2011). "Wakefield's article linking MMR vaccine and autism was fraudulent". *BMJ* 342: c7452.

258. "Vaccine study's author held related patent, medical journal reports". CNN. 11 January 2011. Retrieved 12 January 2011.

259. McKee, Maggie (4 March 2004). "Controversial MMR and autism study retracted". New Scientist. Archived from the original on 13 August 2007. Retrieved 10 August 2007.

260. McCarthy, Jenny (January 10, 2011). "Jenny McCarthy: In the Vaccine-Autism Debate, What Can Parents Believe?". Huffington Post.

261. Sugarman SD. "Cases in vaccine court—legal battles over vaccines and autism". *N Engl J Med*. 2007. 357 (13): 1275–7.

262. McIntyre P, Leask J (2008). "Improving uptake of MMR vaccine". BMJ 336 (7647): 729–30.

263. Justin Norrie. "Japanese measles epidemic brings campuses to standstill". *The Sydney Morning Herald*. May 27, 2007.

264. Molinari NA, Ortega-Sanchez IR, Messonnier ML, Thompson WW, Wortley PM, Weintraub E, Bridges CB. "The annual impact of seasonal influenza in the US: measuring disease burden and costs". *Vaccine*. 2007 Jun 28;25(27):5086-96.

265. Walgreens corporation. "The Impact of a Severe Flu Season: Americans Missed 230 Million Work Days and Lost $8.5 Billion in Wages in 2012-13, Walgreens Flu Impact Report Suggests." October 16, 2013. http://news.walgreens.com/article_display.cfm?article_id=5809.

266. Edwards KM1, Burns VE, Allen LM, McPhee JS, Bosch JA, Carroll D, Drayson M, Ring C. "Eccentric exercise as an adjuvant to influenza vaccination in humans." *Brain Behav Immun*. 2007 Feb;21(2):209-17. Epub 2006 Jul 7.

267. Gretchen Reynolds. "Boosting Your Flu Shot Response With Exercise" *The New York Times* "Well" section. January 16, 2013.

268. Bancos S, Bernard MP, et al. "Ibuprofen and other widely used non-steroidal anti-inflammatory drugs inhibit antibody production in human cells." *Cell Immunol*. 2009; 258(1): 18-28.

269. Woolston. Chris. "You sweat, but toxins likely stay." *The Los Angeles Times*. January 28, 2008.